MARSHA HECKMAN, CATHY OBIEDO & CLAUDIA ALLIN

Illustrations by Jane Kurisu

A LINDA SUNSHINE BOOK

HOW TO CUT YOUR OWN HAIR

(or Anyone Else's!)

THIS BOOK IS DEDICATED TO JACKSON AND TO BERNIE BROOKLYN, BECAUSE BABIES AND PUPPIES ARE THE ONLY THINGS WE LOVE MORE THAN A GREAT HAIR DAY.

Copyright © 2008 Black Dog & Leventhal Publishers, Inc.

All rights reserved. No part of this book, either text or illustration, may be used or reproduced in any form without prior written permission from the publisher.

Published by
Black Dog & Leventhal Publishers, Inc.
151 West 19th Street
New York, NY 10011

Distributed by
Workman Publishing Company
225 Varick Street
New York, NY 10014

Manufactured in China

Cover and interior design by ohioboy art & design

Cover photo, of Austyn Trombold, by Marsha Heckman.

Illustrations copyright © 2008 Jane Kurisu

ISBN-13: 978-1-57912-592-9

h g f e d c b a

Library of Congress Cataloging-in-Publication Data available upon request.

Table of Contents

PREFACE 3

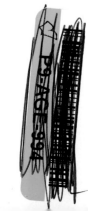

SETTING GELS

For people with very short hair, or for setting your hair on rollers or in pin curls, you don't need to buy commercial setting gel or lotion to hold the set, give your hair volume, or make the curl last longer. Here are some natural alternatives:

1. After washing, towel dry your hair well, then pour beer on your hair and comb it through before setting.

2. If you don't have any beer, dissolve a heaping teaspoon of sugar in four ounces of warm water, and apply the mixture to damp hair before setting. (Don't worry: when the hair is dry, it will not attract bees or ants!)

3. You can make a really effective and healthy setting lotion from flaxseeds. Boil one cup of water and add three tablespoons of flaxseeds. Turn down the heat and simmer, stirring constantly until it reaches the consistency of raw egg white. Strain the mixture, and comb it through damp hair as a setting lotion. Refrigerate the remaining lotion for future use.

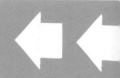

Hair Care for Swimmers

* Before swimming, apply a little oil to the dry ends to protect them from chemicals, salt and the sun.

* Shampoo chlorine or salt water out of your hair soon after swimming. If you can't shampoo right away, at least rinse with cool water.

* A great way to remove swimming-pool chemicals from your hair is by rinsing it with beer.

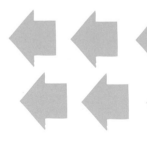

"CLEAN UP COMPLEXION, SOFTEN EYE LINES, SOFTEN SMILE LINE, ADD COLOR TO LIPS, TRIM CHIN, REMOVE NECKLINES, SOFTEN LINE UNDER EARLOBE, ADD HIGHLIGHTS TO EARRINGS, ADD BLUSH TO CHEEK, CLEAN UP NECKLINE, REMOVE STRAY HAIR, REMOVE HAIR STRANDS FROM DRESS, ADJUST COLOR AND ADD HAIR ON TOP OF HEAD, ADD DRESS ON SIDE TO CREATE BETTER LINE . . . TOTAL: $1,525." —INVOICE FOR RETOUCHING THE COVER PHOTO OF MICHELLE PFEIFFER IN THE DECEMBER 1990 ISSUE OF *ESQUIRE* MAGAZINE, OBTAINED BY HARPER'S. THE PHOTO'S CAPTION READS "WHAT MICHELLE PFEIFFER NEEDS . . . IS ABSOLUTELY NOTHING."

"IF TRUTH IS BEAUTY, HOW COME NO ONE HAS THEIR HAIR DONE IN THE LIBRARY? " —Lily Tomlin

PREFACE

We are three sisters who grew up together in San Francisco, California. My sisters, Cathy and Claudia, cut hair for a living, and I am a writer.

Cathy opened her salon, Cambiar (Hair Changes), twenty-nine years ago in northern California, and it is truly a family business. Claudia works at Cambiar with Cathy's son, Paul, and my daughter, Wendy. While my sisters are busy cutting, styling and coloring hair, I can usually be found at the flower market. I am the author of four books, all with how-to components, encouraging readers to do their own weddings and flower arrangements and even instructing them on how to make beautiful Hawaiian flower leis.

A few months ago, our editor approached us to create a book that would show readers how to cut their own (or anybody else's) hair at home. She knew we were the perfect team for the job. We've always been an artistic family, and we love to work on creative projects together. Cathy, Claudia and I were excited to take on this challenge and share our knowledge gained from years of doing hair.

This book will help you become even more self-sufficient than you already have to be in our fast-paced and increasingly expensive world. Do-it-yourself haircutting will keep your style updated and save you money and time between appointments with your favorite haircutting professional. Cutting your and your family's hair can be fun and can give you a true feeling of accomplishment too. You can experiment with new looks or just do maintenance trimming to keep your style neat and fresh. You may find that cutting your child's hair is an enjoyable activity.

Share this book with a friend and use it as a guide to cut each other's hair, or at the very least ask him or her to help you with the back of your own haircut. Save time and money by learning how to trim your own bangs or clean the neckline of your husband's hair.

We feel good about sharing inside information for cutting and caring for your hair, and we hope you have as much fun doing it as we have had writing about it. The illustrations in this book, by the multitalented Jane Kurisu, provide easy-to-follow, step-by-step directions to make any cut that much easier to accomplish.

We encourage you to experiment and be bold with those scissors. Remember, your hair grows half an inch every month, or six inches a year, so whatever you do, your hair will replace itself, giving you a chance to refine your style or try another look entirely.

—Marsha Heckman, Cathy Obiedo & Claudia Allin
August 2007

"PEOPLE ALWAYS ASK ME HOW LONG IT TAKES TO DO MY HAIR. I DON'T KNOW. I AM NEVER THERE. " —Dolly Parton

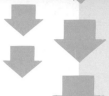

NATURAL CONDITIONERS

1. Flaxseed oil from the health-food store or gourmet food market is a soothing emollient conditioner that softens dry hair. It can also be used as a styling agent for long or short hair—men's, kids' or women's. Just apply and comb through damp hair.

2. The gel of the aloe vera plant is a wonderful natural conditioner that soothes and softens dry or damaged hair. Cut the aloe leaf lengthwise, scoop out the fleshy gel, and push it through a strainer. Apply the strained gel to clean, towel-dried hair, and distribute it through your hair with a wide-tooth comb. Cover your hair with a plastic bag for at least ten minutes, then lightly rinse. The older the aloe vera plant, the more healing properties it contains.

3. Use lemon juice or apple cider vinegar diluted with water as a rinse to remove any build up of natural oils, dirt and hair products.

4. A few drops of rosemary oil is an excellent treatment for combating dryness and taming frizz and split ends, as well as providing shine. Sprinkle this fine oil on your hairbrush and brush through dry hair, paying attention to covering the driest parts. Hair will absorb the oil, and because the molecules are tiny, it won't leave your hair feeling or looking greasy.

TEA TIME FOR YOUR HAIR

Herbal teas are good for your hair. Some of the most popular and effective include:

Rosemary, for dryness and enhancing the color of brown and black hair

Comfrey, for shine and dryness

Walnut leaves, to darken hair

Chamomile, to enhance and highlight blonde hair

Sassafras and a little **saffron,** to highlight red hair

Mint and **eucalyptus** leaves, for itchy, dry scalp

Nettles and **rosemary,** for dandruff and other scalp problems

To prepare the tea, pour two cups of boiling water over a quarter cup of dried herbs. Cover, steep until cool, and strain the herbs. Pour tea over clean, dry hair. Catch the overflow in a bowl, and reapply several times for best results. Rinse hair with cool water.

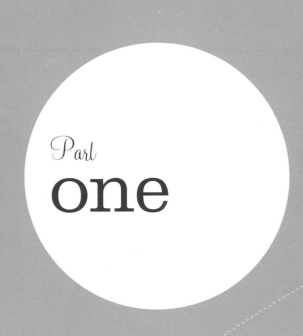

Part
one

GETTING STARTED

"THE THREE MOST IMPORTANT THINGS
TO A SOUTHERN GIRL ARE GOD, FAMILY AND HAIR,
ALMOST NEVER IN THAT ORDER. **"** —*Lucinda Ebersole,*
The New York Times Magazine, 1990

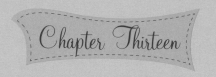

Chapter Thirteen

"I THINK THE LONGER I LOOK GOOD, THE BETTER GAY MEN FEEL."

—*Cher*

NATURAL HAIR CARE PRODUCTS

Using natural treatments for your hair is like eating nutritious food for your body. Many commercial products contain dyes, preservatives and alcohol that can contribute to dryness and damage your hair. You risk using detergent and other chemicals when you buy cheaper products at the grocery store or drugstore. The best commercial products are found only in hair salons. They are more likely to contribute to healthy hair, and are selected and tried by professionals.

You can easily make healthy concoctions in your kitchen that rival the effects of commercial hair care products of all kinds: flaxseed oil for styling gel, sugar water as mousse, cactus for conditioner, herbs to treat dandruff. These inexpensive, natural ingredients are easy to find and make much healthier hair treatments. Give some of these traditional recipes for your hair a try.

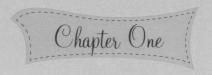

Chapter One

FIND YOUR BEST STYLE

Most women choose a hairstyle from a photo of a favorite celebrity, or a model in a style book, or a magazine at the hair salon. Current fashion should not be your only criteria; if you have short, dark, curly hair, you can't realistically expect to look like Jennifer Aniston or Reese Witherspoon. Of course, you may be able to replicate Oprah's 'do if you have expensive hair extensions and a team of stylists at your beck and call.

Instead of copying others, look at your own face and decide what would work best for you. Be guided by the shape of your face. Hair is like a frame that can disguise unflattering angles. Hair can also emphasize and highlight your best features, like those killer cheekbones or big, baby blue eyes. To accomplish the most flattering cut, you must also consider the texture of your hair. Everyone's hair—curly, straight, thick or thin—can be beautiful if treated with the right products and cut to the best advantage. Let's start with the shape of your face.

Part *five*

HAIR CARE

"I USE MANE 'N TAIL SHAMPOO THAT I GET FROM THE EQUESTRIAN CENTER. THINK ABOUT IT—LOOK AT HORSES WITH THEIR LONG, SMOOTH, SILKY MANES." —*Jennifer Aniston,* *Us Weekly, November 5, 2001*

HOW TO DETERMINE THE SHAPE OF YOUR FACE

The most important first step is to determine the shape of your face. This is easy: stand close to your mirror, hair pulled back, and draw the outline of your face with an erasable marker or that lipstick you never wear. Step out of the frame of the mirror, and the shape of your face will be staring back at you.

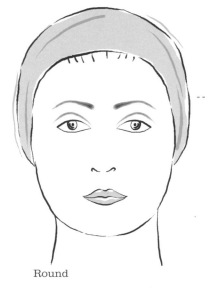

Round

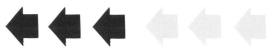

Round face: Play down the roundness of this face by giving yourself some height at the crown of your head. Keep the sides of your hair close to your head, or make them longer to create the illusion of length in your face. Longer hair allows you to wear your hair up. Shaggy or wispy sides are also flattering. Bangs should be straight in the center of your forehead and a little longer on each side.

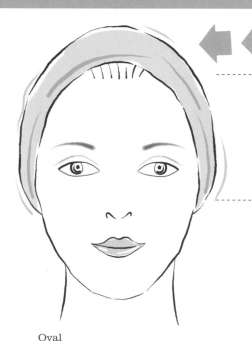

Oval

Oval face: In our culture, the oval face is considered the most pleasing and symmetrical. If your face is oval, most any haircut will work well. If not, our advice is to find a style that will make your face appear to be oval.

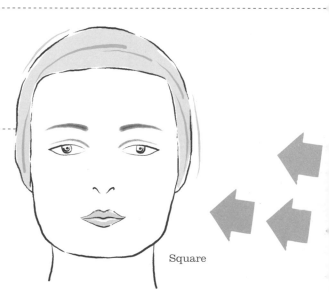

Square

Square face: Flatter the square face by minimizing the angles of your forehead and jawline with your hairstyle. Waves or curls that fall at the sides of your forehead, asymmetrical bangs, or a side part will achieve this. Long layers that start just above your jaw and lie softly around the sides of your face will complement a square shape. An angular bob is not for you.

step 16
WHEN YOU REACH THE EAR, MAKE ANOTHER ONE-INCH SECTION, FROM THE EAR UP TO THE CENTER OF THE FRONT.

step 17
COMB THE HAIR STRAIGHT OUT FROM THE SCALP.

step 18
CUT TO THE SAME LENGTH AS THE SECTION BEHIND THE EAR.

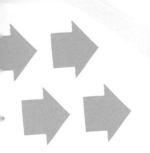

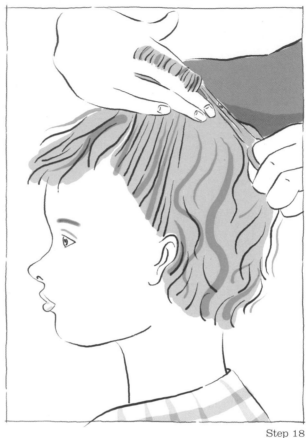

Step 18

step 19
REPEAT ON THE OTHER SIDE.

step 20
COMB THE WHOLE HEAD OF HAIR INTO PLACE, AND NEATLY CUT AROUND THE EARS.

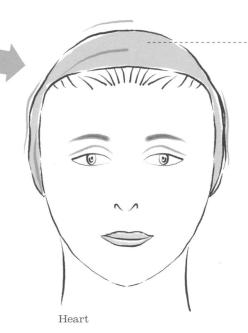

Heart

Heart-shape face: A heart-shape face is defined as narrower at the chin with a wide forehead. The most flattering cut for this shape is shoulder-length hair that is full or softly layered on the sides, lying close to your face at the top. Short sides tend to make a heart-shape face look even wider. Cutting your bangs along the contour of your eyebrows minimizes the width of your forehead. Added fullness at your chin and fringe-style bangs will balance the heart shape.

Diamond or oblong face: A diamond or oblong face is approximately one-half as wide as it is long. Proper length is important to make your face look more proportionate. Shoulder-length hair, with substantial bangs that cover the narrowest part of the forehead, is good for an oblong face, and side layers that brush the cheeks add width. It's best not to cut your hair shorter than chin length. If you want longer hair, create bangs or a side part, and angle the cut from your cheekbones.

Oblong

BASIC HAIR CARE FACTS

* To keep your hair looking healthy, eat a lot of vegetables and foods high in vitamin A, vitamin C, vitamin B, iron, iodine and copper.

* Hair grows on average a quarter- to a half-inch a month, and this process slows down dramatically as you age.

* Hair does not turn gray with age; it actually loses color due to the lack of new color pigment in each strand of hair.

* Overbleached hair does not shine because the outer layer, or cuticle, is lifted and no longer reflects light.

* Only the tiniest molecules can penetrate the hair's cuticle. The smallest molecules of any oil are in the kukui nut, from the tropics.

* When cutting your own hair, don't worry if you make a mistake—a professional can always fix your blunders. And remember, hair grows back!

step

13 MAKE A ONE-INCH SECTION FROM THE CROWN TOWARD THE NECK, PULLING THE HAIR STRAIGHT OUT FROM THE SCALP.

step

14 CUT THIS SECTION OF HAIR, MATCHING THE LENGTH TO THE TOP SECTION.

step

15 MAKING VERTICAL SECTIONS PARALLEL TO THE SECTION YOU JUST CUT, CONTINUE CUTTING TO MATCH EACH SECTION TO THE LENGTH OF THE SECTION NEXT TO IT.

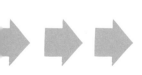

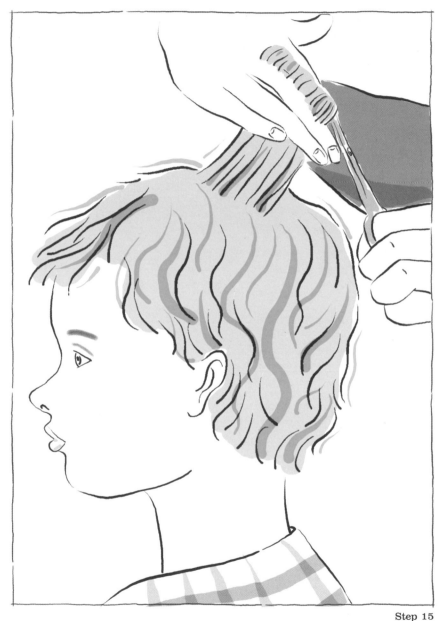

Step 15

HAIR TEXTURE AND THE APPROPRIATE CUT

Fine, straight hair: A blunt cut, all one length, usually works best for straight, fine hair. The now-classic Sassoon cut that is shorter in back and grazes the jawline in front is ideal for fine, straight hair. Whether you choose to have bangs depends on the shape of your face.

Thin hair: A short, textured cut makes any hair type look thicker. A choppy cut or curls, with proper use of a good volumizing product, is most becoming.

Thick hair: Rely on your face shape to guide you lucky ones with thick hair. If your hair is straight, a variation of a long or short bob will always work. Thick, curly hair should be shaped well when cut short. It's also great worn long with combs, barrettes, headbands or ribbons, and can be made elegant when slicked back into a bun or braid.

Curly or kinky hair: It is best to layer very curly hair to avoid too much volume that can swallow your face. This is better than torturing your hair every day with straighteners or heat. Length should be determined by the shape of your face and the style that complements your features.

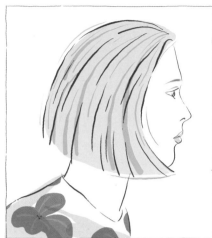

Fine, straight hair

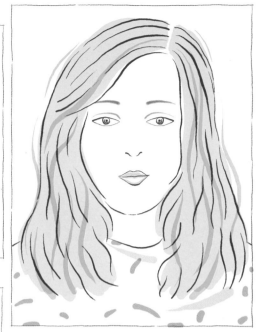

Thick hair

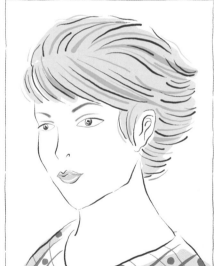

Thin hair

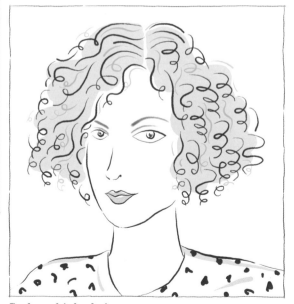

Curly or kinky hair

step

10

PART THE HAIR INTO A SECTION AN INCH WIDE, FROM THE FOREHEAD TOWARD THE CROWN.

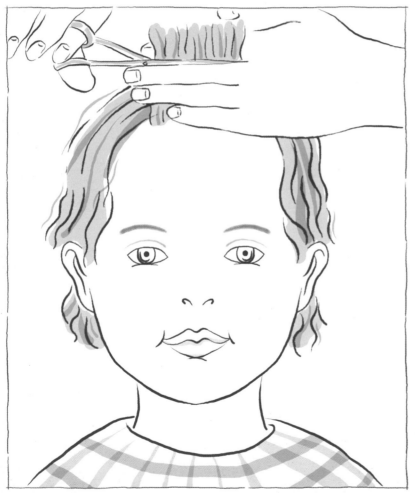

Step 11 & 12

step

11

COMB THE HAIR STRAIGHT UP FROM THE SCALP, GRASPING IT BETWEEN YOUR INDEX AND MIDDLE FINGERS.

step

12

CUT THIS SECTION TO THE LENGTH YOU WANT.

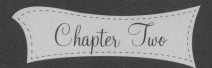
Chapter Two

"I'M A BIG WOMAN. I NEED BIG HAIR."

—*Aretha Franklin*

WHAT YOU NEED TO CUT HAIR

Before picking up those scissors, decide exactly what you want to do. Pick a style, and stick to it. Changing your mind mid-cut can be a problem, as after you cut, the hair is gone for now. So be realistic and plan ahead. It is probably best not to do anything extreme, at least at first. If you have long hair and want to make it short, cut it in gradual steps, a little bit at a time. Wait until you feel really comfortable with the scissors before making a radical change.

First, look at yourself in the mirror. What exactly do you want to accomplish? Do you want to keep your same hairstyle, but a bit shorter? Even the ends or cut off damaged hair? Get your bangs out of your eyes?

Next, read the appropriate chapter instructions. This book will give you all the information you need to cut your hair, but it is best if you read through the entire chapter before you begin.

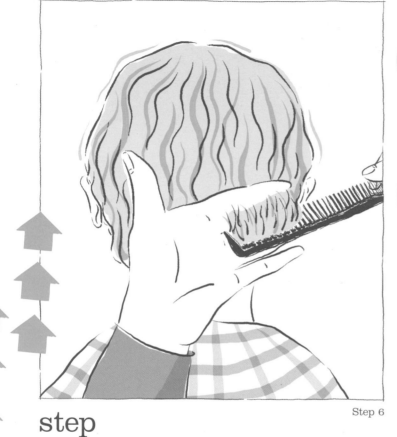

Step 6

step

8 CUT ON AN ANGLE FROM THE CENTER OF THE EAR TO THE CENTER OF THE NECK IN BACK.

step

9 REPEAT ON THE OPPOSITE SIDE. YOU'VE NOW ESTABLISHED THE PERIMETER OF THE CUT.

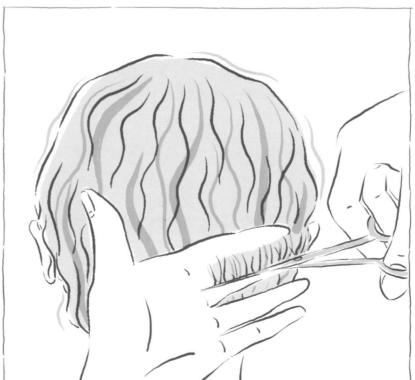
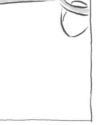

Step 8

step

6 PICK UP THE SECTION OF HAIR BEHIND THE EAR, AND COMB IT FROM UNDERNEATH.

step

7 GRASP THE SECTION OF HAIR BETWEEN YOUR INDEX AND MIDDLE FINGERS.

TOOLS OF THE CUT

To cut hair, you need the right tools. Find each tool on our list, and place it in front of you before you start to cut.

Here is what you will need:

1. Sharp scissors or clippers—dull scissors will not cut hair well

2. Rat-tail comb for sectioning

3. Spray bottle of water to keep hair damp while you cut

4. Combs
   a. wide-tooth comb for long hair and thick hair
   b. fine-tooth comb for short hair and fine hair

5. Half a dozen hair clips (use jaw-style clips for long hair)

6. Two mirrors—a wall mirror and a handheld mirror, to check the back

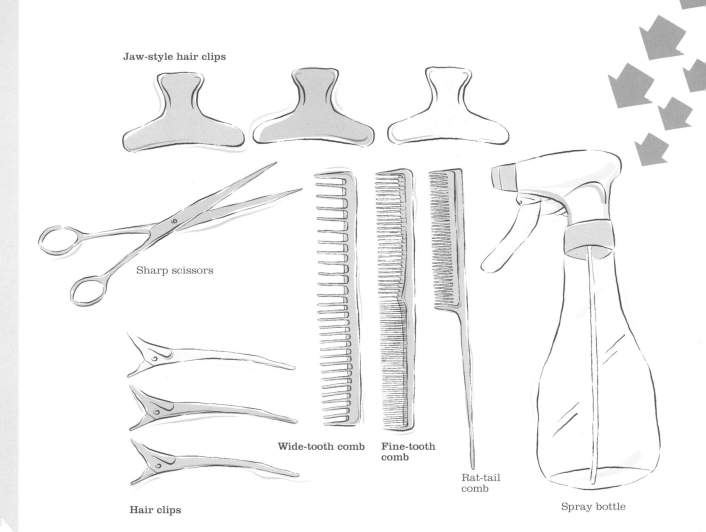

Jaw-style hair clips

Sharp scissors

Hair clips

Wide-tooth comb

Fine-tooth comb

Rat-tail comb

Spray bottle

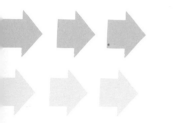

step

3 START IN THE FRONT, COMBING AND GRASPING A SECTION OF HAIR ON ONE SIDE OF THE PART BETWEEN YOUR INDEX AND MIDDLE FINGERS.

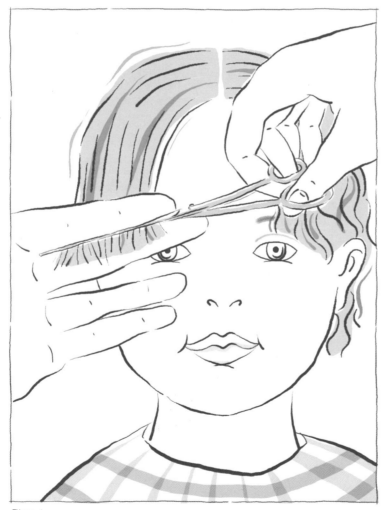

Step 4

step

4 CUT ON AN ANGLE FROM THE EYEBROW TOWARD THE MIDDLE OF THE EAR.

step

5 REPEAT ON THE OPPOSITE SIDE.

Prepare to Cut Your Hair

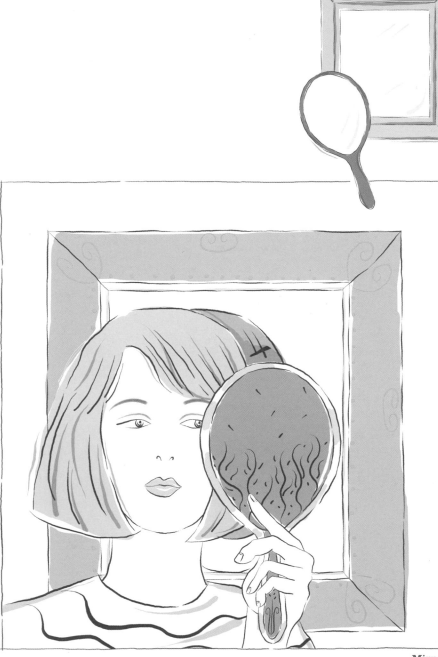

Mirrors

* Once you have read through the proper chapter and have a good idea of what you intend to accomplish, wash and condition your hair as normal. (See page 12 for the best way to shampoo your hair.)

* Leave your hair wet. You may want to tuck a hand towel or dishtowel into your collar to keep cut hairs from scratching your neck.

* In front of the mirror, section your hair according to the instructions and secure it with clips.

* Read the instructions one last time, and go for it.

KIDS' SHORT HAIR

step 1
PART THE CHILD'S HAIR DOWN THE CENTER.

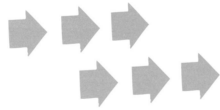

step 2
COMB THE HAIR STRAIGHT DOWN ON THE SIDES.

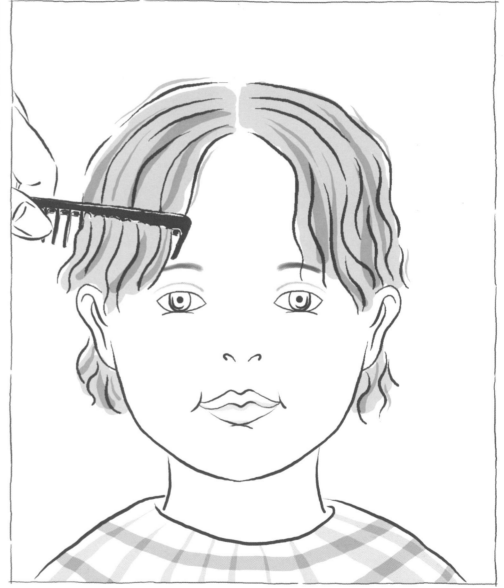

Step 1 & 2

Shampoo Secrets

* When washing your hair, use only a dab of shampoo. (If you do not generate enough lather, add a little more water, not shampoo.) A small bit will go a long way, and the less you use, the less residue you leave on your hair. Too much shampoo also strips natural oils and contributes to split ends and flyaway hairs.

* When shampooing, scrub your hair at the scalp, where oil and dirt build up. Shampoo will go through the hair well enough to clean it without you having to scrub the ends.

* After washing, always rinse your hair with very cool water, which closes the cuticles and allows hair to maintain body and shine.

* Always blot hair dry, never rub. Rubbing creates tangles which can cause spilt ends. Massage products into your hair.

* There's no right answer to how often you should wash your hair, as it varies for each person. You know best when you need to wash your hair. Wash hair daily if you want to as long as you use quality products.

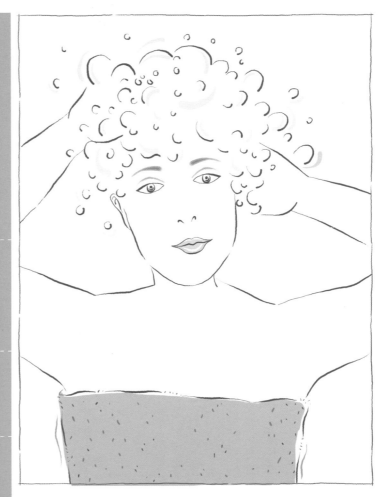

❝ I'D LOVE TO KISS YA', BUT I JUST WASHED MY HAIR. ❞ —*Bette Davis*

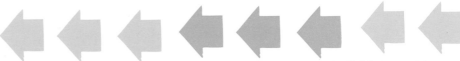

step

7

CONTINUE CUTTING ACROSS THE FRONT TO THE OPPOSITE
SIDE, MATCHING THE LENGTH AS YOU WORK.

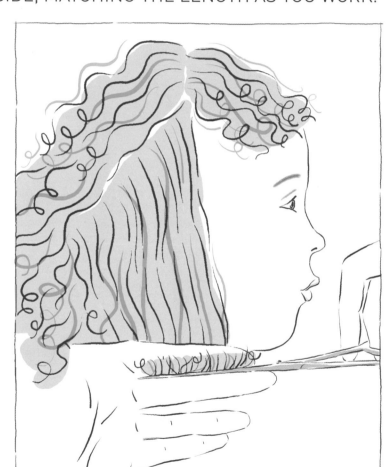

Step 7

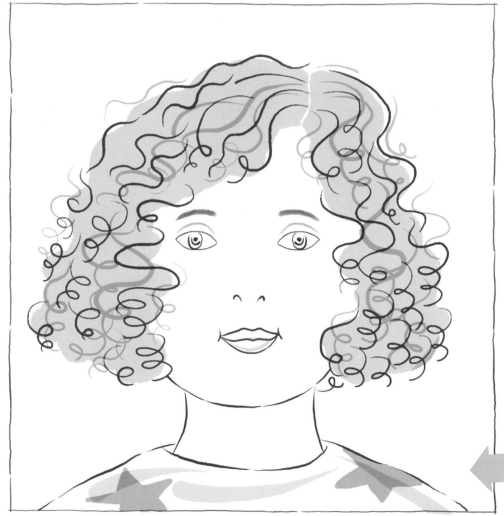

Final long, curly cut

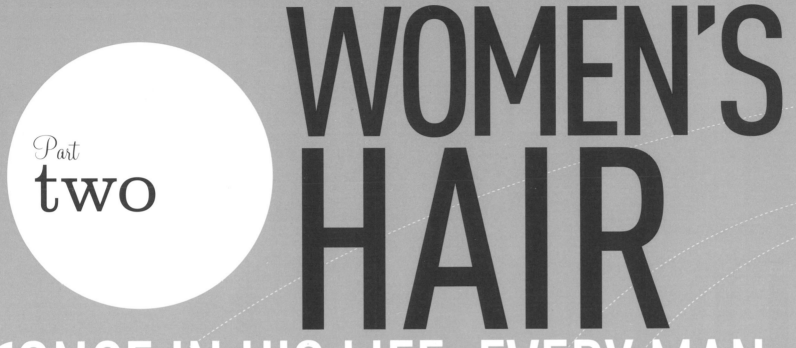

WOMEN'S HAIR

"ONCE IN HIS LIFE, EVERY MAN IS ENTITLED TO FALL MADLY IN LOVE WITH A GORGEOUS REDHEAD. " —*Lucille Ball*

step 4

COMB THE BACK FROM THE CROWN
STRAIGHT DOWN ONTO THE NECK.

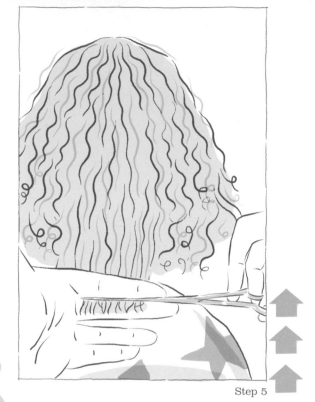

Step 5

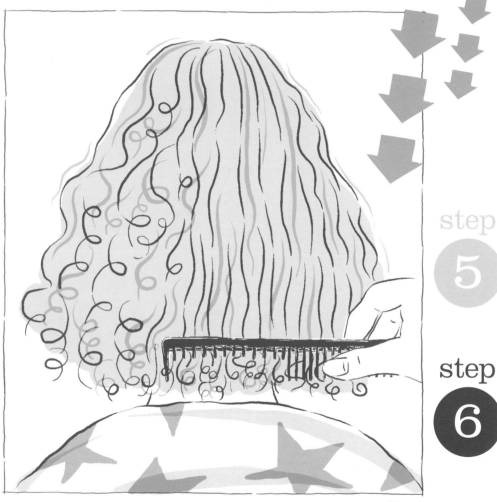

Step 4

step 5

STARTING AT THE BACK, GRASP A SECTION OF HAIR
WITH YOUR INDEX AND MIDDLE FINGERS JUST ABOVE
WHERE YOU WANT TO CUT, PULLING THE HAIR TAUGHT
TO STRAIGHTEN THE CURL, AND CUT.

step 6

REMINDING THE CHILD TO HOLD STILL, COMB ONE SIDE
SECTION. AGAIN, CREATING ENOUGH TENSION TO PULL
OUT THE CURL, CUT A STRAIGHT LINE JUST UNDER YOUR
FINGERS, MATCHING THE FIRST CUT.

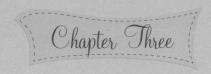

Chapter Three

HOW TO CUT YOUR BANGS

"MY HUSBAND SAID HE WANTED TO HAVE A RELATIONSHIP WITH A REDHEAD, SO I DYED MY HAIR."

—*Jane Fonda*

The word "bangs" comes from *banga*, an ancient Norse word meaning "to hammer." The word evolved to signify a sudden or abrupt sound or movement. By the nineteenth century, "bang-on" had become an English expression meaning direct and abrupt, and cutting a bit of hair straight and quickly across the forehead was cutting your hair "bang off." Because the British call bangs "fringe," it's possible the American use of "bangs" came from a horse-grooming term, "bangtail," where the end of the equine tail is cut neatly squared off.

KIDS'
LONG, CURLY HAIR

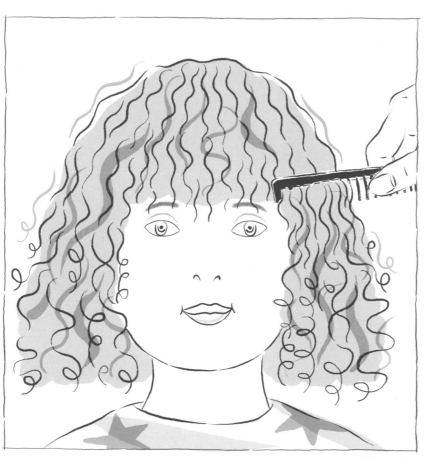

Step 2 & 3

step 1
IF THERE ARE BANGS, CUT THEM FIRST AS INSTRUCTED IN THE PREVIOUS SECTION. (REMEMBER, CURLY HAIR WILL SPRING BACK AND LOOK SHORTER, SO CUT OFF LESS HAIR.)

step 2
COMB THE CHILD'S HAIR FORWARD FROM THE CROWN OF THE HEAD TOWARD THE FOREHEAD.

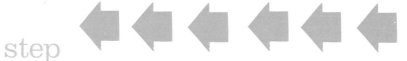

step 3
COMB THE SIDES STRAIGHT DOWN OVER THE EARS.

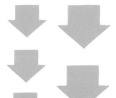

Depictions of ancient Egyptians show both royalty and slaves alike wearing bangs. Most upper-class hair arrangements were actually wigs, but common people wore bangs to keep their hair out of their eyes while working. In modern times, bangs became popular in the 1920s, when women began bobbing their hair. There are lots of women who hide behind their bangs (or hide an unattractive hairline or extremely high forehead) and would never do away with them, no matter what fashion dictates. Learning how to cut bangs can be the first step in learning how to cut hair, and it can save you a lot of money at the hairdresser's. Changing *only* your bangs can give your style a completely different look. And everyone who has ever worn bangs knows how annoying it is when they grow too long.

Bang styles can vary from blunt (thick and straight) to wispy and textured. Your bangs can also be shaped and cut along your eyebrows, or longer on the sides of your face. Because hair grows half an inch a month, bangs need constant maintenance and should be cut about every other week.

The Big Bangs Theory

* Asymmetrical or long, wispy and layered bangs are best for a square face.

* Bangs that are cut blunt and shaped along the contour of the eyebrows will minimize the width of the forehead on a heart-shape face.

* For an oblong or diamond-shape face, cut longer, textured bangs, or sweep them to the side. Have your bangs cover the narrowest part of your forehead.

* Soft and layered bangs, straight in the center of your forehead and a little longer on each side, or longer bangs combed to one side, elongate a round face.

* Any style can work for an oval face, so your priorities should be your hair's texture and the style you prefer.

step 6
REPEAT ON THE LEFT SIDE, MATCHING THE LENGTH TO THE RIGHT SIDE.

step 7
COMB ALL THE HAIR TO THE BACK AND CHECK THAT THE TWO SECTIONS ARE EVEN.

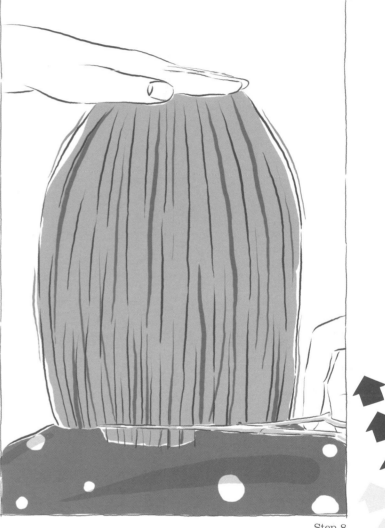

Step 6

Step 8

step 8
WITH ONE HAND ON THE TOP OF THE CHILD'S HEAD, SNIP ANY LONGER HAIRS TO MAKE THE LINE STRAIGHT.

THE TWIST
METHOD

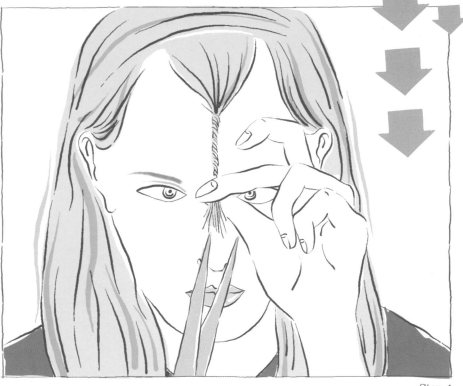

Step 4

step

1 SECTION THE AMOUNT OF HAIR YOU WANT TO CUT OR TRIM AS BANGS.

step

2 COMB THE SECTION TO THE FRONT OF YOUR FACE.

step

3 TWIST AND HOLD THE SECTION IN FRONT OF YOUR NOSE.

step

4 GAUGE THE LENGTH YOU WANT TO CUT, AND GRASP YOUR HAIR BETWEEN YOUR INDEX AND MIDDLE FINGERS, JUST ABOVE THIS LINE.

step

5 HOLD THIS SECTION IN FRONT OF YOUR NOSE TO CENTER IT, AND CUT JUST BELOW YOUR FINGERS.

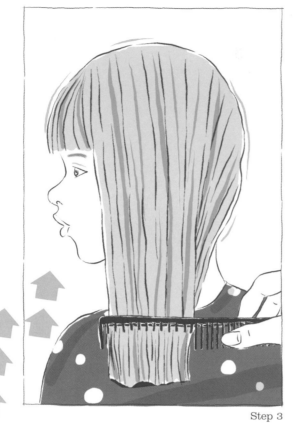

Step 3

step
5
REMINDING THE CHILD TO HOLD STILL, CUT A STRAIGHT LINE JUST UNDER YOUR FINGERS.

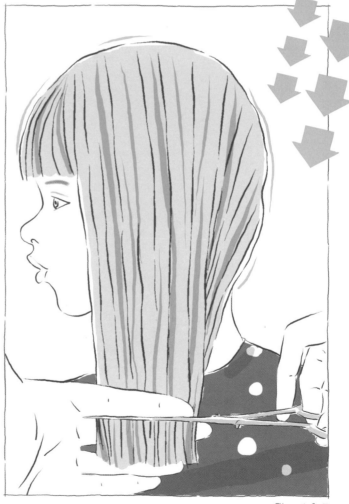

Step 4 & 5

step
3
TELL THE CHILD TO TURN HIS OR HER HEAD ALL THE WAY TO THE RIGHT. COMB THE SECTION STRAIGHT DOWN IN FRONT OF THE SHOULDER.

step
4
GRASP THE HAIR WITH YOUR INDEX AND MIDDLE FINGERS JUST ABOVE WHERE YOU WANT TO CUT.

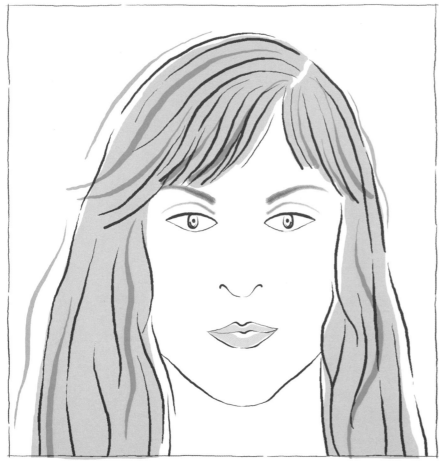
Result of the twist method

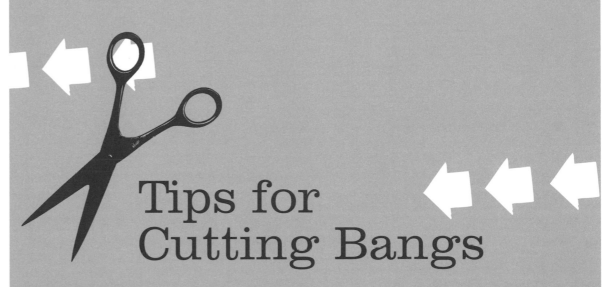

Tips for Cutting Bangs

* When cutting wet bangs, always make them a bit longer than desired, as they will shorten as they dry. You can always cut off more if they end up too long.

* Longer, wispy bangs are versatile and can be combed to the side of your face or back for variety.

* Use a flat iron to straighten bangs, or use a curling iron to bend the ends under for dimension and fullness.

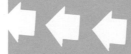

KIDS'
LONG, STRAIGHT HAIR

step

1 CUT THE BANGS FIRST, AS INSTRUCTED ON PAGES 76 TO 78.

step

2 COMB THE CHILD'S HAIR, AND DIVIDE IT INTO TWO SECTIONS, FROM THE CENTER OF THE FOREHEAD TO THE BACK.

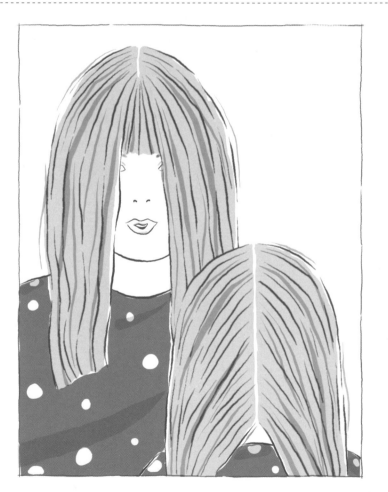

BLUNT BANGS

1 SECTION THE AMOUNT OF HAIR YOU WANT TO CUT OR TRIM AS BANGS, AND PIN THE REST OF YOUR HAIR OUT OF THE WAY.

step

2 HORIZONTALLY DIVIDE THE SECTION INTO TWO THINNER SECTIONS, AND PIN THE TOP SECTION OUT OF YOUR WAY.

step

3 COMB THE BOTTOM SECTION STRAIGHT DOWN, AND HOLD IT BETWEEN YOUR INDEX AND MIDDLE FINGERS.

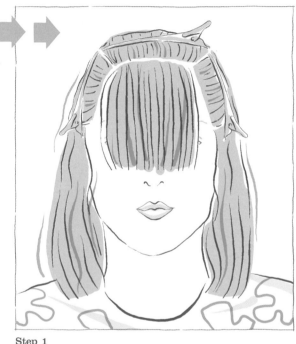

Step 1

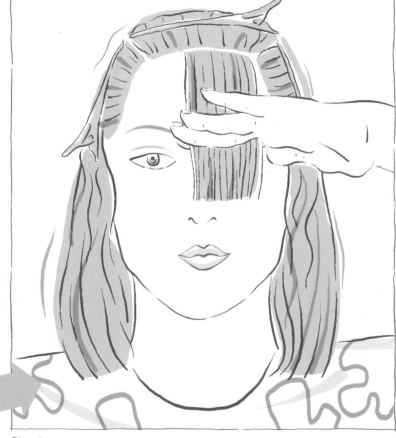

Step 3

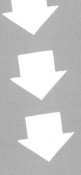

Helpful Tips for Cutting Kids' Hair

* To help keep your child's head still while you cut, have her close her eyes. Kids will automatically turn to look at anyone who talks or anything making a sound. Try saying, "How long can you keep your eyes closed? I'll count while you do it."

* Give little kids their favorite toy, blanket, pacifier, finger food, or drink with a straw.

* Have someone read to them while you are cutting, with the reader in front of the child.

* Tell the child that when his or her hair is cut, it won't make tangles anymore. Comb out the tangles with a leave-in spray conditioner before you cut.

* Some very young children are understandably afraid that cutting hair will hurt. Assure them that cutting hair is *not* like cutting skin. Quickly snip a piece of hair and say, "See, you can't even feel that."

* And don't forget, there's always the all-powerful bribe.

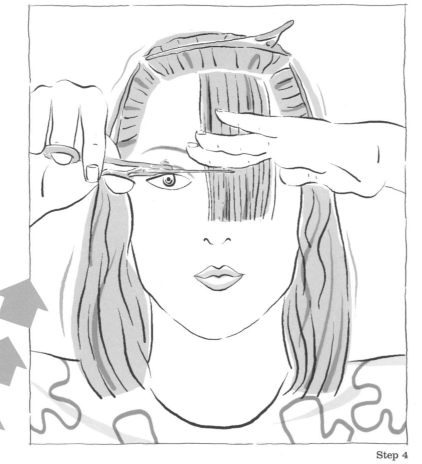

Step 4

step

6 CUT THE LONGER HAIRS TO THE SAME LENGTH AS THE SHORTER ONES.

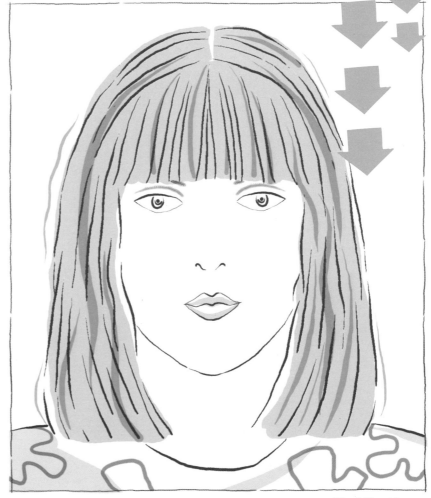

Final blunt bangs

step

4 CUT THE SECTION IN A STRAIGHT LINE ACROSS YOUR FOREHEAD, DIRECTLY BELOW YOUR FINGERS.

step

5 UNPIN AND COMB THE SECOND SECTION WITH THE FIRST, HOLDING BOTH SECTIONS BETWEEN YOUR FINGERS.

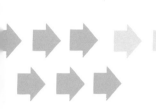

step 6

COMB THE SECOND SECTION TOGETHER WITH THE FIRST, AND CUT THE LONGER HAIR TO MATCH.

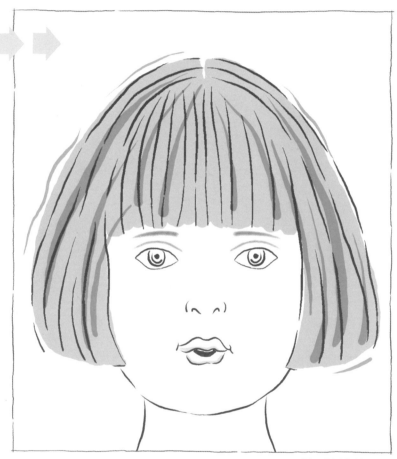

Final kids' bangs

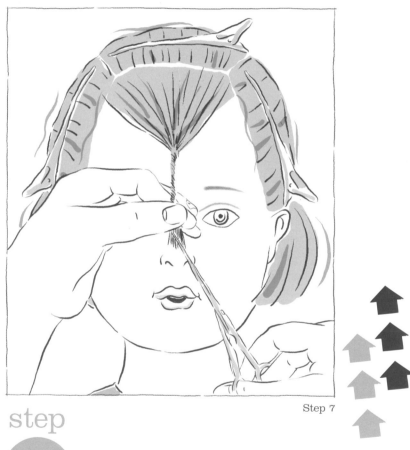

Step 7

step 7

FOR MORE WISPY BANGS, COMB AND TWIST THE BANGS TOGETHER, HOLD THEM IN FRONT OF THE CHILD'S NOSE, AND CUT THEM TO THE DESIRED LENGTH.

SHAPED BANGS

step 1

SECTION THE AMOUNT OF HAIR YOU WANT TO CUT OR TRIM AS BANGS, AND PIN THE REST OF YOUR HAIR OUT OF THE WAY.

step 2

COMB THE SECTION OVER YOUR FOREHEAD.

step 3

CUT THE SECTION WITH SEVERAL SMALL SNIPS OF THE SCISSORS, USING THE SHAPE OF YOUR EYEBROWS AS YOUR GUIDELINE. USE THIS METHOD TO CUT ASYMMETRICAL BANGS, BANGS THAT ARE SHORTER IN THE CENTER, OR ANY SHAPE YOU WANT.

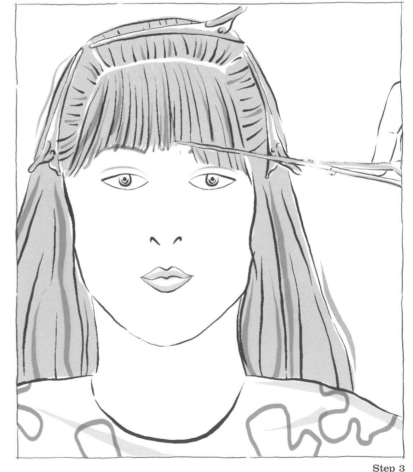

Step 3

step

4 HOLD THE HAIR BETWEEN YOUR INDEX AND MIDDLE FINGERS.

step

5 CUT A STRAIGHT LINE JUST UNDER YOUR FINGERS.

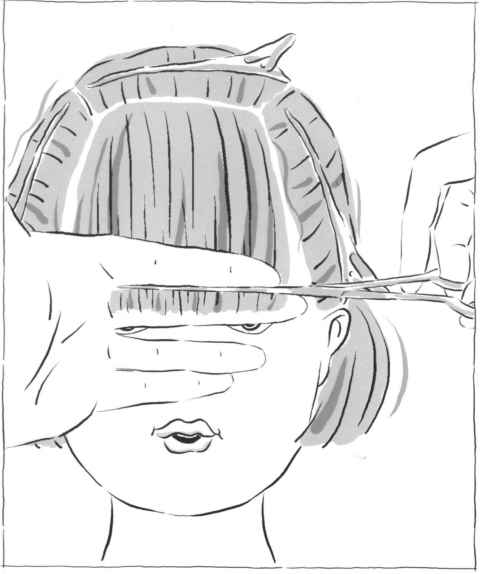

Step 4

WISPY, TEXTURIZED BANGS

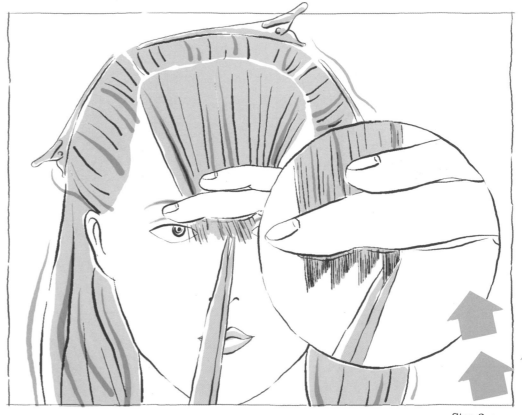

Step 3

step 1

TO CREATE CASUAL, CHOPPY OR WISPY BANGS, FIRST CUT THEM BLUNT, SHAPED OR CONTOURED BY THE TWIST METHOD.

step

COMB AND HOLD THE BANGS HALF AN INCH FROM THE ENDS.

step 3

HOLDING THE SCISSORS PERPENDICULAR TO THE LINE OF THE CUT, CHOP SMALL V-SHAPE SECTIONS.

KIDS' BANGS

step

2 COMB THE SECTION TO BE CUT FORWARD, AND TELL THE CHILD TO CLOSE HIS OR HER EYES.

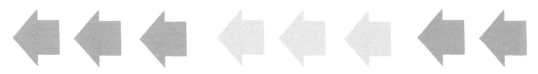

step

3 IF THE BANGS WILL BE THICK, DIVIDE THE HAIR INTO TWO SECTIONS PARALLEL TO THE CHILD'S HAIRLINE. THINNER BANGS CAN BE CUT IN ONE SECTION.

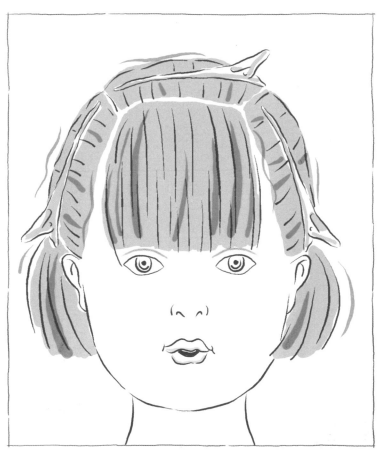

Step 1 & 2

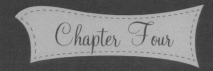

Chapter Four

HOW TO CUT LONG, STRAIGHT HAIR

"LONG HAIR IS CONSIDERED BOHEMIAN, WHICH MAY BE WHY I GREW IT, BUT I KEEP IT LONG BECAUSE I LOVE THE WAY IT FEELS, PART CLOAK, PART FAN, PART MANE, PART SECURITY BLANKET."

—*Marge Piercy*, *Braided Lives*

From Delilah, Rapunzel and Lady Godiva to Angelina Jolie, a long mane of beautiful tresses has always been touted as a woman's crowning glory. Most men love long hair, considering it sexy and youthful. Little girls wear long hair (and cut it off to announce they are grown up). If you've been wearing your hair long and want a real change, cut it, but do it in increments to avoid any regret. It will grow back, but not overnight.

One more thing to remember: the trick to cutting long, straight hair is keeping your head in the same position for the entire cut.

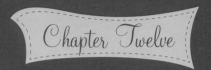

Chapter Twelve

"I USED TO GET A HAIRCUT EVERY SATURDAY SO I WOULD NEVER MISS ANY OF THE COMIC BOOKS. I HAD PRACTICALLY NO HAIR WHEN I WAS A KID!"

—*R. L. Stine*

TRIMMING KIDS' BANGS AND CUTTING HAIR

Cutting your kid's hair, whether curly or straight, long or short, can save you a lot of money and can be a fun experience for both you and your child—if you follow our advice. (It comes from years of haircutting *and* parenting.) You need to deal with their fear and wiggling to get the job done.

Remember to constantly use positive reinforcement: "That's perfect, just like you're doing now. You're holding still better than a grown-up. Good!"

Always start by cutting the perimeter of the hair— bangs and neckline or bottom—in case you aren't able to finish the entire process.

To make the haircutting time as short as possible, do a minimum of sectioning when cutting small children's hair.

Remember, when cutting curly hair, to put the same amount of tension on every section to straighten out the curl, making it even.

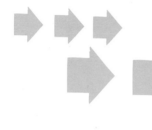

step

1

PART YOUR HAIR INTO TWO SECTIONS, STARTING AT YOUR FOREHEAD AND DRAGGING THE COMB IN A STRAIGHT LINE ALL THE WAY BACK TO YOUR NECK.

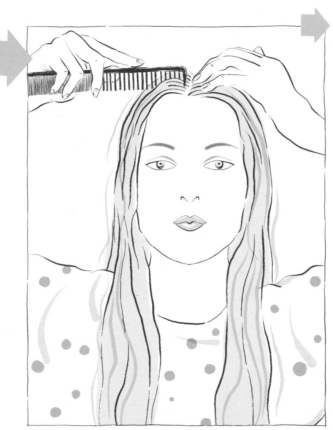

Front

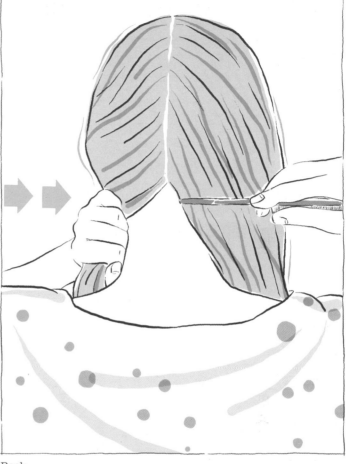

Back

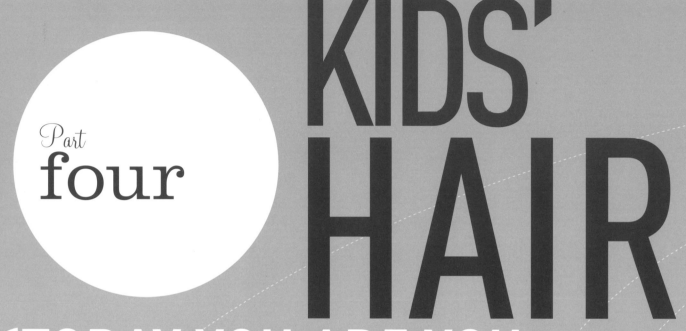

Part
four

KIDS' HAIR

"TODAY YOU ARE YOU, THAT IS TRUER THAN TRUE. THERE IS NO ONE ALIVE WHO IS YOUER THAN YOU." —*Dr. Seuss*

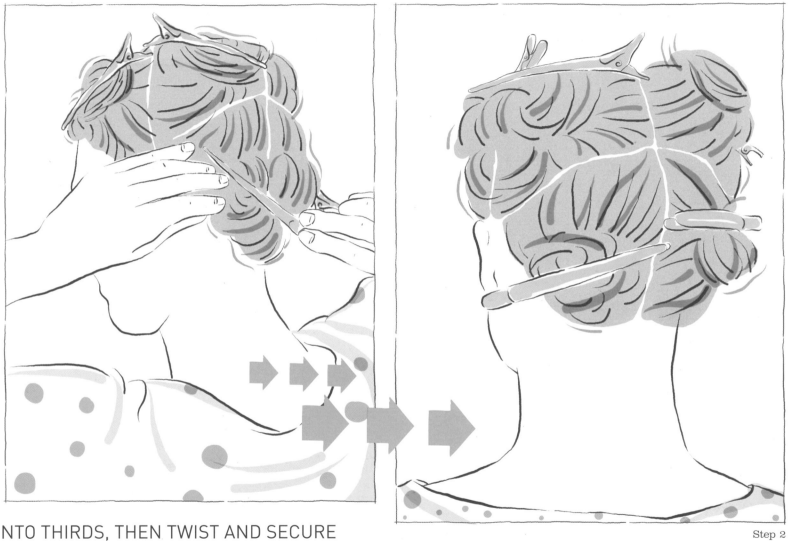

2

PART EACH HALF INTO THIRDS, THEN TWIST AND SECURE
EACH SECTION OF HAIR WITH A CLIP, CLOSE TO YOUR SCALP.

Step 2

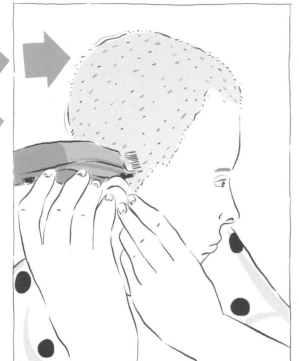

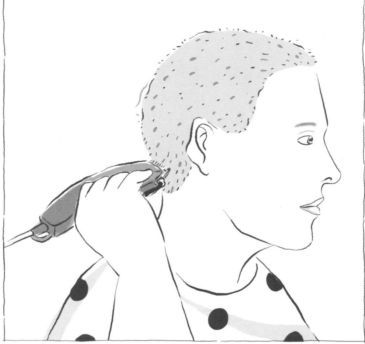

Step 5

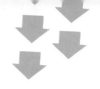

step 6

CHANGE THE GUARD FOR THE OPPOSITE EAR AND REPEAT.

step 7

PUT THE FIRST GUARD YOU USED BACK ON THE CLIPPER, AND GO OVER THE ENTIRE HEAD TO CATCH ANY UNEVEN AREAS.

step 5

CHANGE TO EITHER THE RIGHT OR LEFT EAR GUARD. FOLD THE EAR DOWN, AWAY FROM THE CLIPPER, AND DRAG THE CLIPPER AROUND THE EAR, WITH THE SHORT-TOOTH END OF THE GUARD DOWN. MOVE THE CLIPPER ABOVE THE CUT TO BUZZ THE ENTIRE SIDE.

"HAIR IS THE FIRST THING. AND TEETH THE SECOND. HAIR AND TEETH. A MAN GOT THOSE TWO THINGS, HE'S GOT IT ALL." —*James Brown*

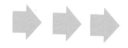

3 TAKE ONE OF THE BACK, BOTTOM
SECTIONS, AND COMB THE HAIR
OVER YOUR SHOULDER.

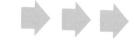

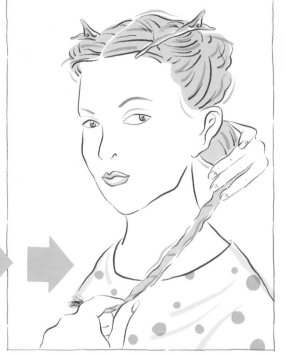

Step 3

step

4 FIRMLY GRASP THE ENDS WITH YOUR FINGERS JUST
ABOVE WHERE YOU WANT TO CUT. (REMEMBER, HAIR
STRETCHES WHEN IT IS WET, SO YOUR HAIR WILL BE A
LITTLE SHORTER WHEN DRY.)

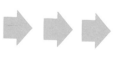

step

5 KEEPING TENSION ON THE HAIR, PINCH THE SECTION
BETWEEN YOUR INDEX AND MIDDLE FINGERS AND CUT
A HORIZONTAL LINE JUST BELOW YOUR FINGERS.

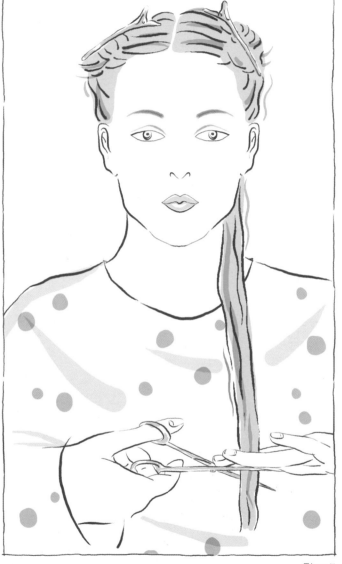

Step 5

step

3

REPEAT ON EITHER SIDE OF THE
CENTER CUT.

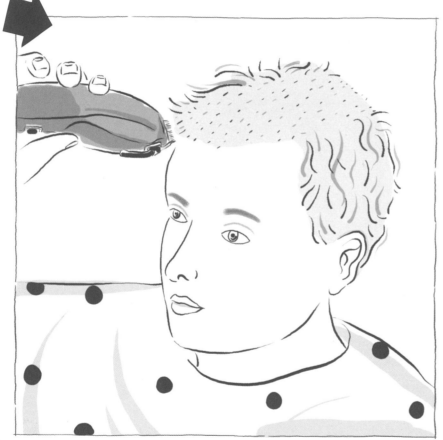

Step 3

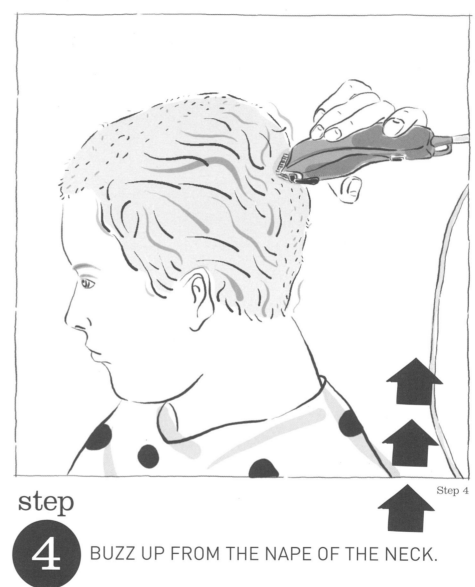

Step 4

step

4

BUZZ UP FROM THE NAPE OF THE NECK.

step 6

UNPIN THE OTHER BACK, BOTTOM SECTION, AND COMB THAT SECTION OF HAIR OVER YOUR OTHER SHOULDER.

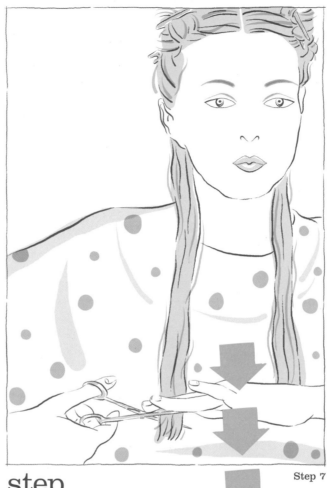

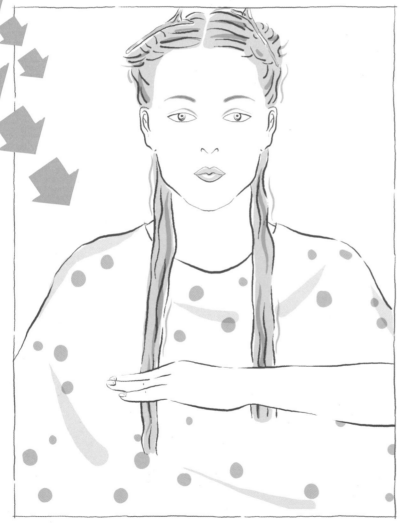

Step 6

Step 7

step 7

FIRMLY GRASP THE ENDS WITH YOUR FINGERS JUST ABOVE WHERE YOU WANT TO CUT, KEEPING YOUR HEAD LEVEL. BE SURE NOT TO TILT YOUR HEAD WHILE CONCENTRATING. LOOK IN THE MIRROR, AND CUT THE LENGTH OF THIS SECTION TO MATCH THE CUT SECTION ON THE OTHER SIDE.

step
1 COMB HAIR AND LEAVE IT DRY.

step
2 START IN THE MIDDLE OF THE HAIRLINE ABOVE THE FOREHEAD. HOLD THE CLIPPER WITH THE GUARD FIRMLY AGAINST THE SCALP, AND SLOWLY DRAG IT ACROSS THE HEAD TOWARD THE BACK.

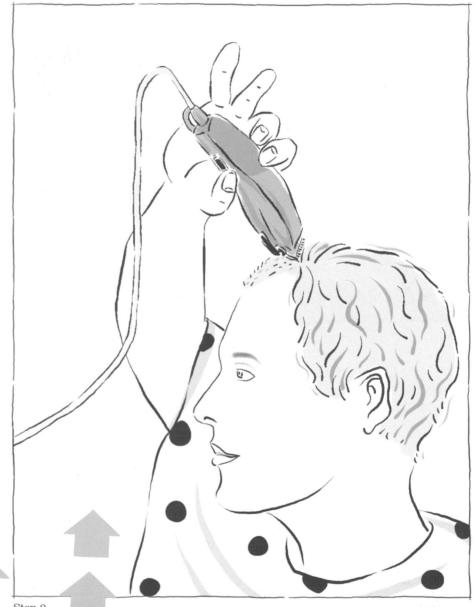

Step 2

step

8

KEEPING YOUR HEAD LEVEL, LOOK IN THE MIRROR (NOT DOWN AT YOUR HAIR!). UNPIN AND COMB THE RIGHT, MIDDLE SECTION STRAIGHT DOWN. HOLD IT WITH YOUR FINGERS EVEN TO THE LINE OF YOUR FIRST CUT ON THIS SAME SIDE.

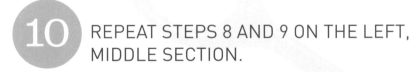

step

9

CUT THIS SECTION.

step

10

REPEAT STEPS 8 AND 9 ON THE LEFT, MIDDLE SECTION.

step

11

UNPIN AND COMB THE RIGHT, FRONT SECTION DOWN, AND HOLD IT WITH YOUR FINGERS EVEN TO THE LENGTH YOU HAVE ALREADY CUT.

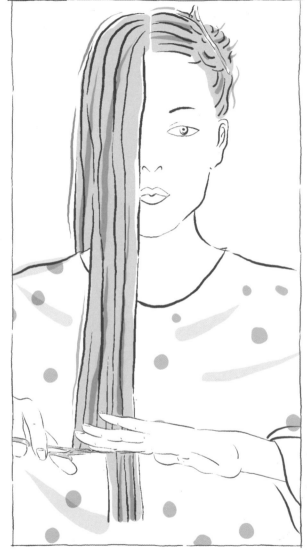

Step 12

step

12

CUT THIS SECTION.

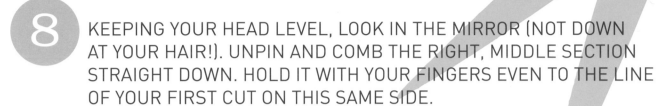

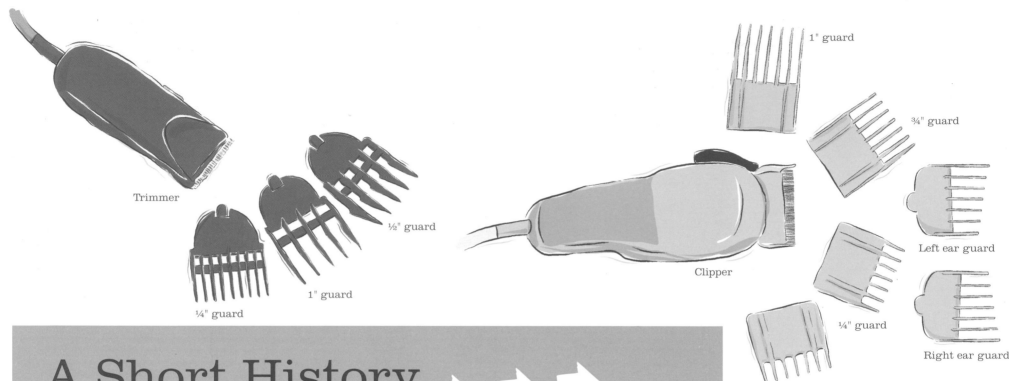

Trimmer

¼" guard

1" guard

½" guard

Clipper

1" guard

¾" guard

Left ear guard

Right ear guard

¼" guard

½" guard

A Short History of Hairdressing

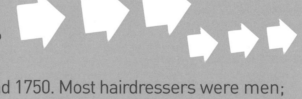

Hairdressing formally became a profession around 1750. Most hairdressers were men; many were trained as wigmakers. The most famous was Legros de Rumigny, who began his career as a baker and became the official hairdresser to the French court of Louis XV. He published the *Art de la Coiffure des Dames* in 1765 and opened Academie de Coiffure, the first beauty college, in 1769.

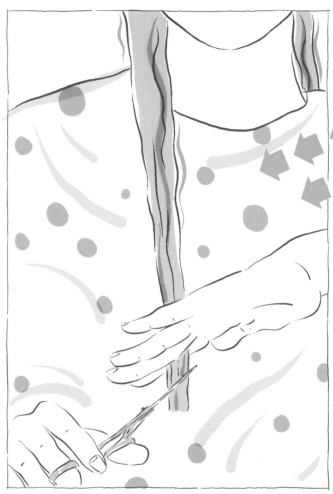

Step 13

step 13

COMB THROUGH THE RIGHT SIDE, AND CHECK THAT ALL YOUR CUTS MATCH. (IF YOU WANT THE FRONT A BIT SHORTER, HOLD THIS SECTION OF HAIR AT AN ANGLE, WITH YOUR FINGERS POINTING AWAY FROM YOUR CHIN, THEN CUT ON A UPWARD ANGLE TOWARD YOUR CHIN.)

step 14

REPEAT STEPS 11, 12, AND 13 ON THE FRONT, LEFT SIDE.

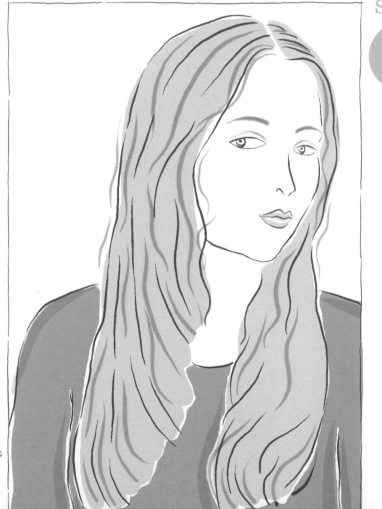

Final angled front

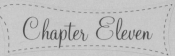

Chapter Eleven

THE
BUZZ CUT

"ANY MAN OVER 30 WITH LONG HAIR LOOKS LIKE HIS MOTHER."

—*Orson Welles*, *Newsweek*, July 30, 1973

With an electric hair clipper, there are a number of guards, usually numbered one through four. These are used to buzz the top and back of the hair. The smaller the number, the shorter the hair will be. A kit will also include guards for each ear that you can use on the sides of the head.

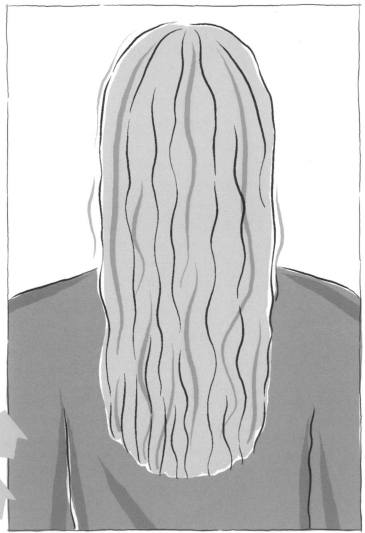

Final long, straight cut / Back

step

15 COMB THROUGH YOUR HAIR, AND USE A HANDHELD MIRROR TO CONFIRM THAT THE BACK IS EVEN.

step

16 COMB THE FRONT TWO SECTIONS FORWARD, AND CHECK THAT THE SIDES AND FRONT ARE EVEN.

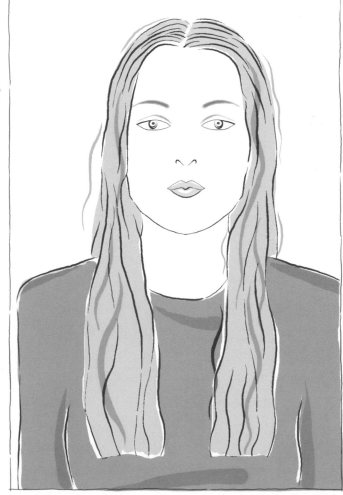

Final long, straight cut

"A HAIR ON THE HEAD IS WORTH TWO ON THE BRUSH." —*Irish Proverb*

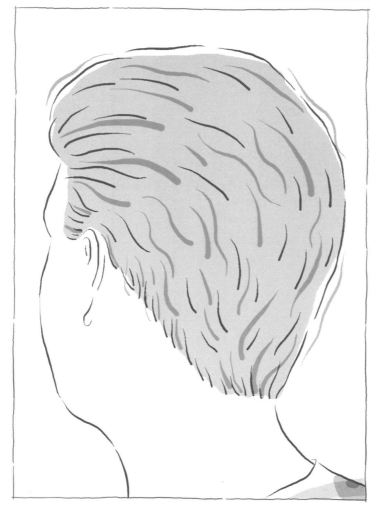

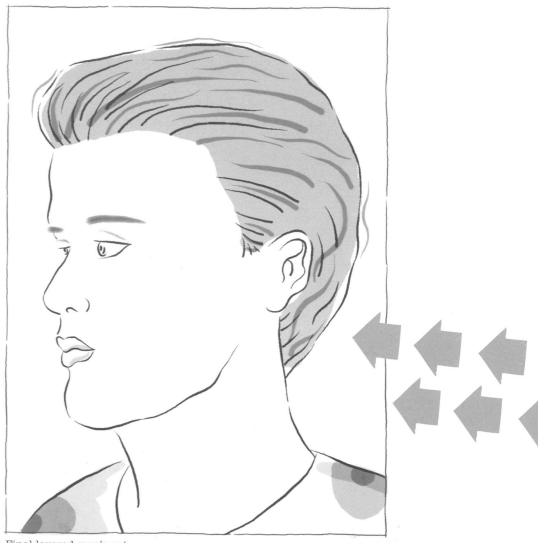

Final layered men's cut

All About Blondes

"GENTLEMEN PREFER BLONDES, BUT GENTLEMEN MARRY BRUNETTES."

—Anita Loos, Gentlemen Prefer Blondes

"I'M NOT OFFENDED BY ALL THE DUMB BLONDE JOKES BECAUSE I KNOW THAT I'M NOT DUMB. I ALSO KNOW THAT I'M NOT BLONDE."

—Dolly Parton

"IT IS POSSIBLE THAT BLONDES ALSO PREFER GENTLEMEN."

—Mamie Van Doren

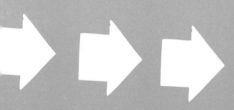

"WHEN YOU'RE NOT BLONDE AND THIN, YOU COME UP WITH A PERSONALITY REAL QUICK."

—Kathy Najimy

"MY REAL HAIR COLOR IS KIND OF A DARK BLONDE. NOW I JUST HAVE MOOD HAIR."

—Julia Roberts

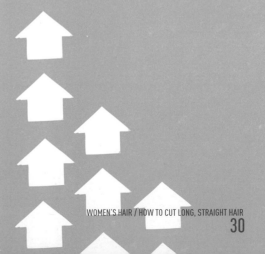

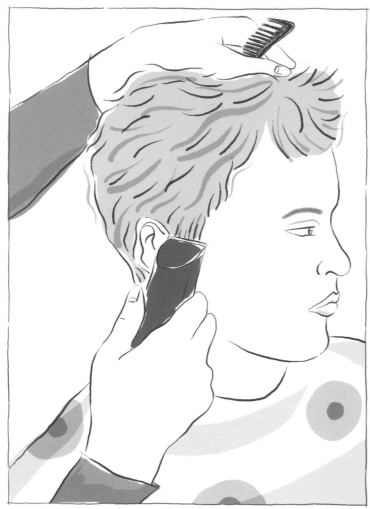

Step 16

step

16

CLEAN UP THE ENDS OF THE SIDEBURNS AND BACK OF THE NECK BY LAYING THE EDGE OF A TRIMMER AGAINST THE SKIN AND PULLING IT STRAIGHT DOWN.

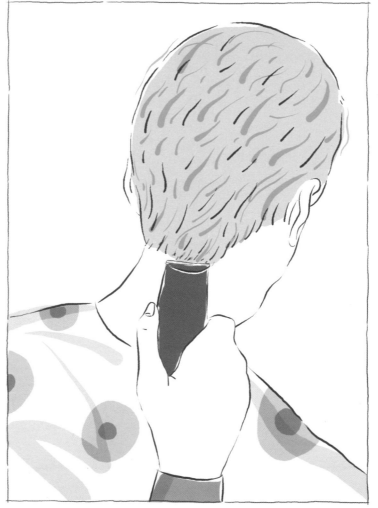

Step 16

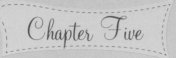
Chapter Five

HOW TO CUT LONG, CURLY HAIR

There are two tricks to cutting long, curly hair: the first is to determine the length you want, then cut off less; the second is to use enough tension to pull out the curl before using the scissors.

Look at your current haircut, and judge how much shorter you want to go. Keep this in mind: the weight of your hair pulls curls down, so the more you cut, the curlier it will be. Once length is cut off, the curls will spring up. If you want the style to look an inch shorter, for example, cut off only a half to three-quarters of an inch.

13
CONTINUE CUTTING UNTIL YOU MEET THE TOP SECTION.

step
14
REPEAT STEPS 9 THROUGH 14 ON THE OPPOSITE SIDE.

step
15
COMB THROUGH THE HAIR, SLIDING IT BETWEEN YOUR INDEX AND MIDDLE FINGERS, AND CUT ANY LONG PIECES OR UNEVEN SECTIONS TO MATCH THE GUIDELINE.

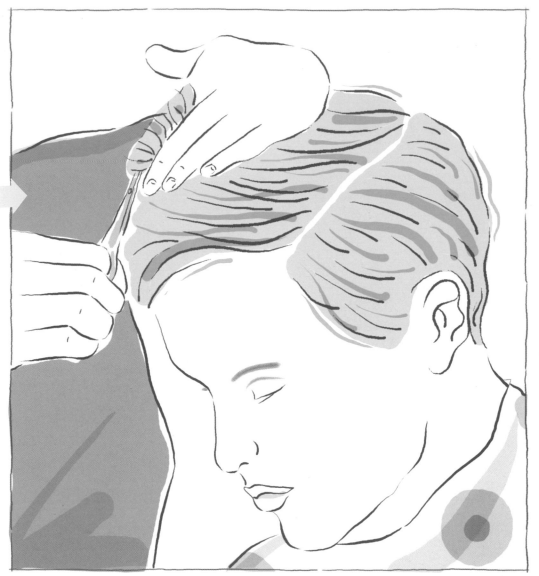

Step 13

1 BEGIN BY FOLLOWING STEPS 1 AND 2
FOR SECTIONING LONG, STRAIGHT HAIR.

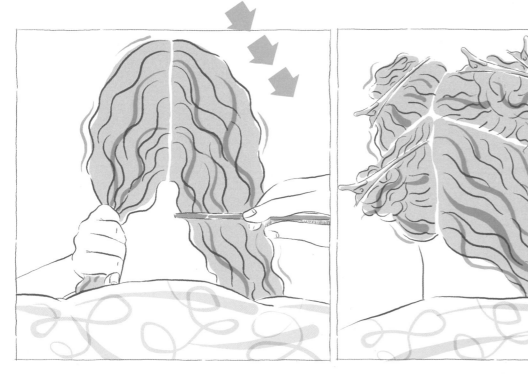

Step 1

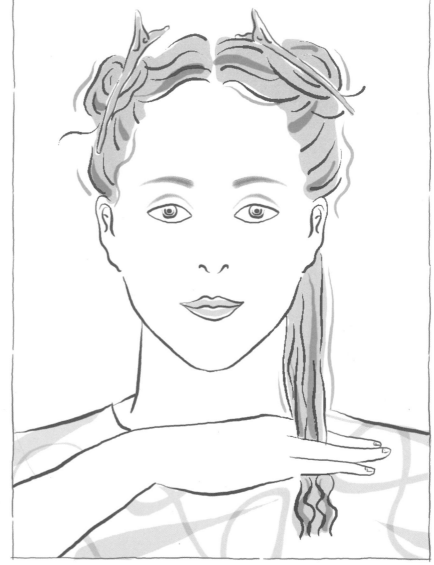

step

2 UNPIN AND COMB EACH SECTION, HOLDING THE HAIR
BETWEEN YOUR FINGERS WITH ENOUGH TENSION
TO PULL THE CURL STRAIGHT. PULLING THE CURL
STRAIGHT ENABLES YOU TO MAKE AN EVEN CUT.

Step 2

step 10

COMB THE FRONT OF THE SIDE FORWARD TOWARD THE TEMPLE, AND CUT AT AN ANGLE TOWARD THE BOTTOM OF THE EAR.

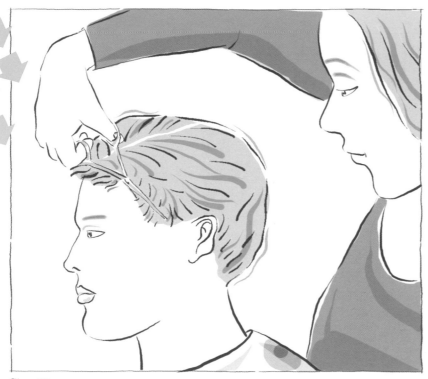

Step 10

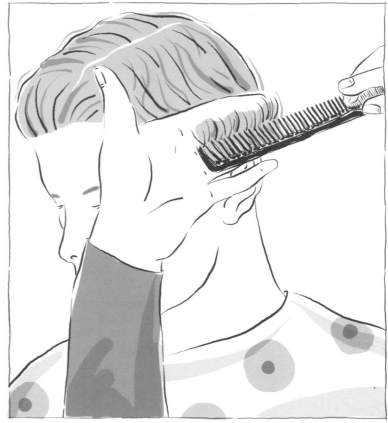

Step 11

step 11

COMB THE HAIR ABOVE THE EAR, PULLING IT OUT.

step 12

GRASP THE UNCUT HAIR WITH YOUR FINGERS, AND CUT IT TO MATCH THE LENGTH OF THE SECTION UNDERNEATH.

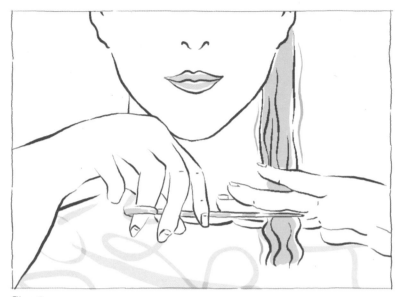

Step 3

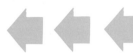 step

3 CUT BELOW YOUR FINGERS IN A STRAIGHT LINE.

 step

4 CONTINUE THROUGH EACH SECTION, APPLYING THE SAME DEGREE OF TENSION AND CUTTING AND MATCHING THE LENGTH TO THE SECTION YOU PREVIOUSLY CUT, UNTIL EVERY SECTION IS DONE.

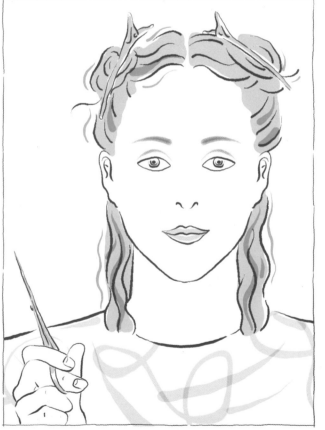

Step 4

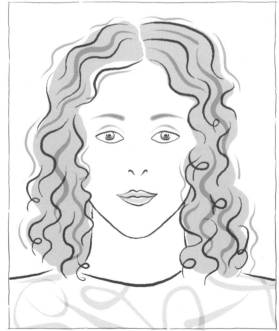

Final long, curly cut

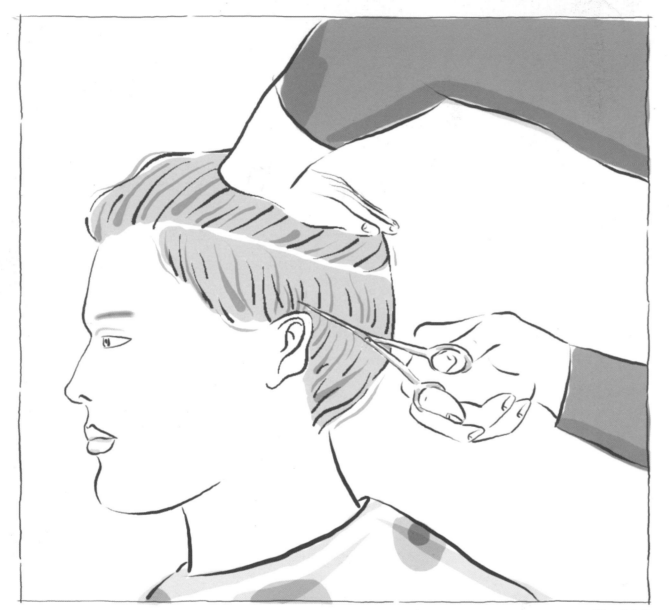

Step 8 & 9

step 8

PART THE HAIR HORIZONTALLY ABOVE THE EAR INTO A ONE-INCH SECTION.

step 9

CUT AROUND THE EAR, CONNECTING TO THE GUIDELINE AT THE BACK.

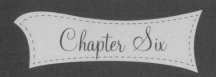

Chapter Six

HOW TO CUT SHORT, STRAIGHT HAIR

Since the 1920s, when women began cutting their hair to show their independence, the bob has been a classic hairdo. In the 1960s, hair guru Vidal Sassoon refined the cut with geometric precision, and the bob thereafter became known as a "Sassoon." (It still is!)

There are many variations to this cut: with or without bangs, parted on the side or in the center; longer in the back or the front, stick-straight or curled under into a long pageboy or a short Prince Valiant. One point is clear: the bob never goes out of style.

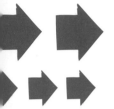

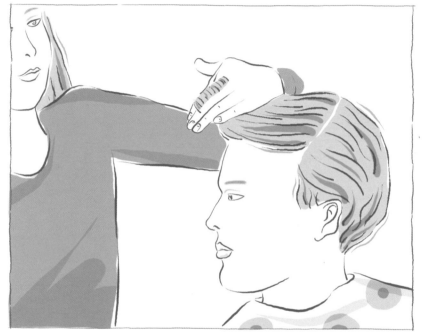

Step 5

5 NEXT, CUT THE FRONT (YOU WILL JOIN THE FRONT AND BACK WHEN YOU CUT THE SIDES). COMB THE HAIR FORWARD, AND GRASP IT BETWEEN YOUR INDEX AND MIDDLE FINGERS.

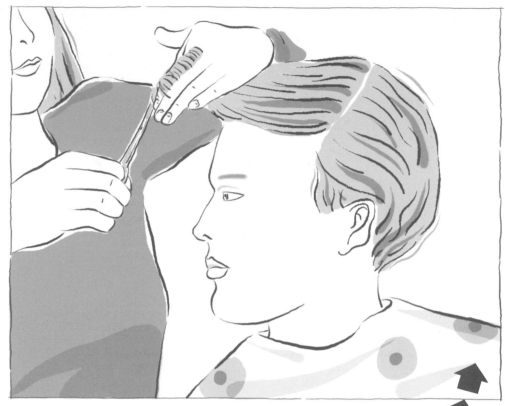

Step 6

step

6 CUT TO DESIRED LENGTH.

step

7 USING THIS CUT AS YOUR GUIDE, COMB ONE-INCH SECTIONS AND MAKE SUCCESSIVE CUTS AS YOU MOVE TOWARD THE BACK.

step 1

COMB HAIR STRAIGHT BACK INTO A PONYTAIL ABOUT AN INCH ABOVE YOUR NECKLINE, AND SECURE WITH A RUBBER BAND.

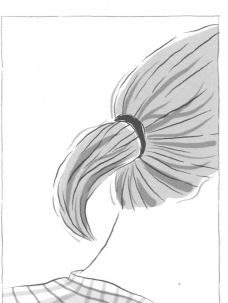

Step 1

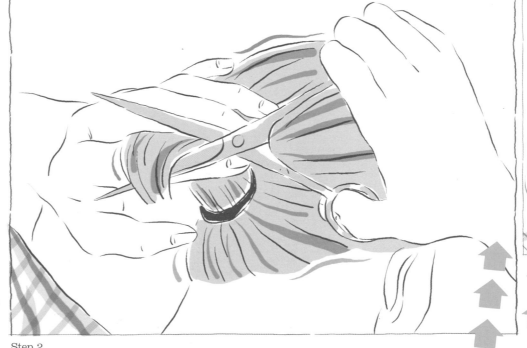

Step 2

Final short, straight cut

step 2

USE A HANDHELD MIRROR TO LOOK AT THE PONY TAIL, THEN GRASP IT IN A STRAIGHT LINE WITH TWO FINGERS BELOW THE RUBBER BAND. PUT THE MIRROR DOWN AND CUT JUST UNDER YOUR FINGERS. YOU MAY NEED TO SNIP SEVERAL TIMES IF YOUR HAIR IS THICK. PUT THE SCISSORS DOWN AND USE THE HAND MIRROR TO CHECK THAT YOUR LINE IS STRAIGHT AND EVEN.

step 3

COMB THE HAIR IN BACK OVER TO THE RIGHT SIDE, AND CUT ON AN ANGLE TOWARD THE EAR. (ULTIMATELY, YOU WILL CREATE A LINE THAT WRAPS FROM THE NAPE OF THE NECK, UP ONE SIDE, ACROSS THE FRONT, AND OVER THE OPPOSITE SIDE.) THIS LINE IS YOUR GUIDE TO CUT THE REST OF THE HAIR THE SAME LENGTH EVENLY.

step 4

REPEAT ON THE OTHER SIDE.

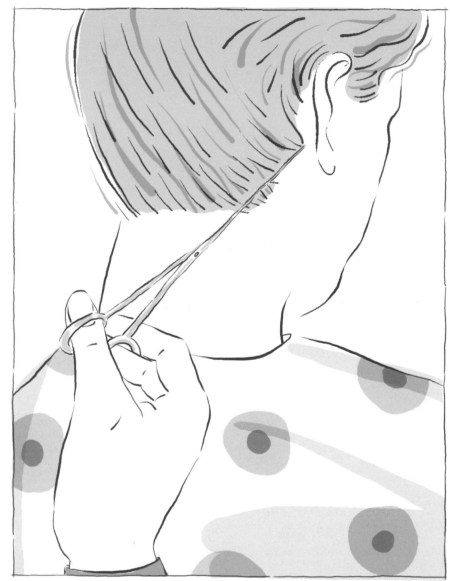

Steps 3 & 4

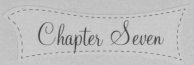

Chapter Seven

HOW TO
CUT LAYERS

"I GET A LOT OF CRACKS ABOUT MY HAIR, MOSTLY FROM MEN WHO DON'T HAVE ANY."

—Ann Richards

A layered cut can make your hair fuller and give it more body. Your hair will stand away from your scalp and frame your face more softly than a one-length style. You can keep your hair long and layer it to remove damaged ends, which will make your hair healthier and shinier.

step

1 GET THE HAIR WET, AND COMB THROUGH.

step

2 CUT THE BOTTOM BACK STRAIGHT ACROSS THE NECKLINE AT THE LENGTH YOU WANT.

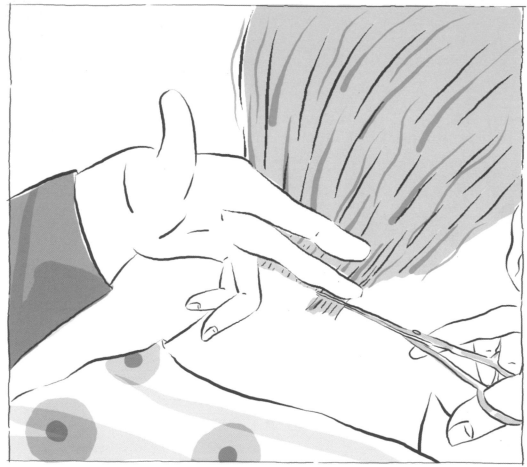

Step 2

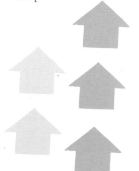

step

 2 COMB THIS SECTION OF HAIR FORWARD.

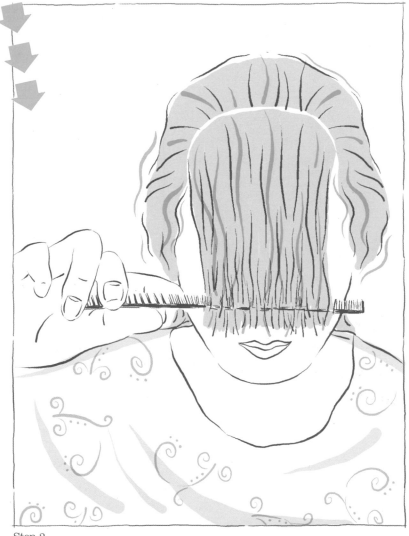

Step 2

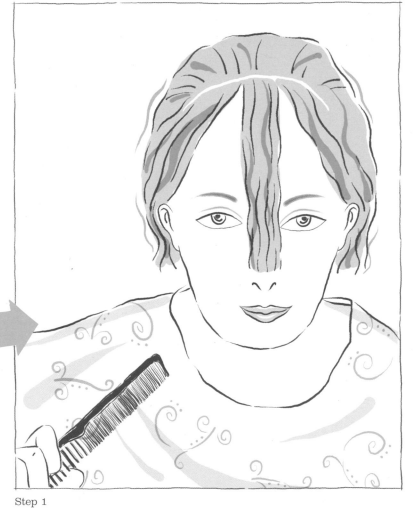

Step 1

 step

1

MAKE A PART AT YOUR HAIRLINE ABOVE THE INNER END OF YOUR EYEBROW ON ONE SIDE, THEN ABOVE THE OPPOSITE EYEBROW. MAKE THIS SECTION AN INCH THICK. (COMB THE SIDE SECTIONS STRAIGHT DOWN, OR TUCK THEM BEHIND YOUR EARS, OUT OF THE WAY.)

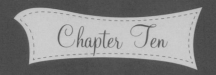

Chapter Ten

THE LAYERED
MEN'S CUT

Do you want to just use a trimmer to neaten up a man's or boy's neckline and sideburns between haircuts at the unisex salon or barbershop? Are you ready to give your guy the full cut?

All you need are these directions, good tools and patience. The goal is to create a neat and even length on the sides and back, with a flattering amount of hair on top. These directions will work on straight or curly hair, and you can cut to any length desired by you (or him).

step

3 GRASP THE HAIR BETWEEN YOUR INDEX AND MIDDLE FINGERS AT THE LENGTH YOU WANT.

step

4 CUT A STRAIGHT LINE JUST UNDER YOUR FINGERS. THIS CUT DETERMINES THE LENGTH OF THE TOP LAYERS.

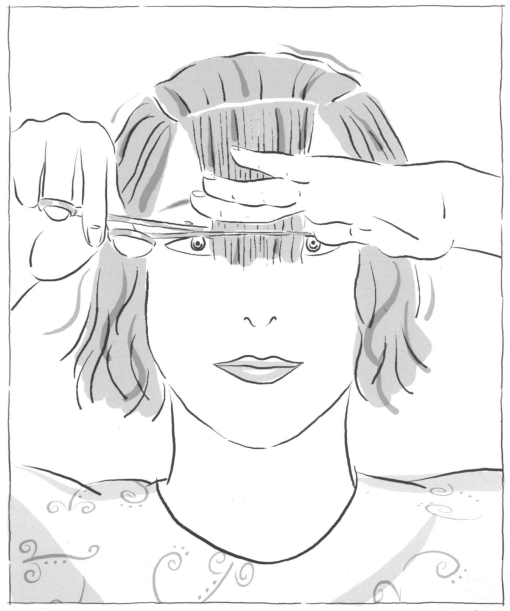

Step 4

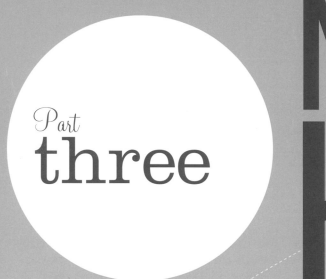

Part
three

MEN'S HAIR

"TOO BAD THE ONLY PEOPLE WHO KNOW HOW TO RUN THE COUNTRY ARE BUSY DRIVING CABS AND CUTTING HAIR." —*George Burns*

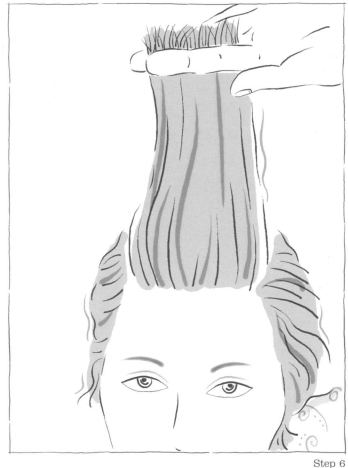

Step 6

step

5

WITH A COMB, MAKE ANOTHER ONE-INCH SECTION BEHIND THE SECTION YOU JUST CUT.

step

6

COMB ALL THE HAIR IN THIS SECTION STRAIGHT UP.

step

7

USING THE SECTION YOU JUST CUT AS A GUIDE, CUT THE NEW SECTION TO THE SAME LENGTH.

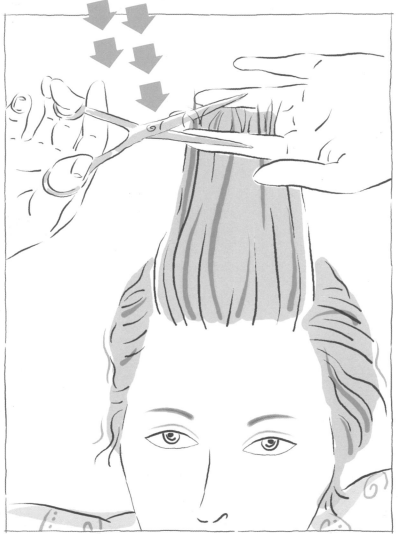

Step 7

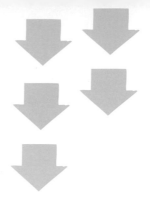

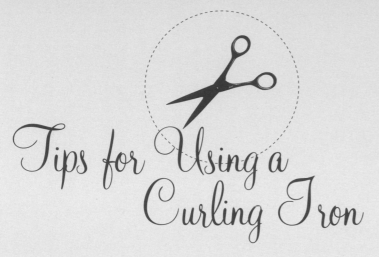

Tips for Using a Curling Iron

* Curling irons come in different sizes. Choose one with a diameter that will give you the curl size you desire.

* Divide your hair into sections, and begin curling from the back, bottom section, working up toward the front, top section.

* Make thicker sections for waves and soft curls, and thinner sections for tighter, springy curls.

* Always curl your hair in small, manageable sections, as if setting it on rollers.

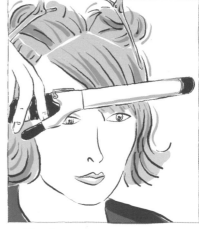

curling bangs

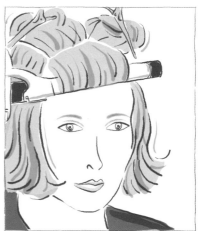

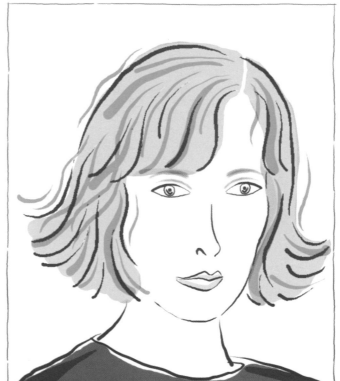

Final curling iron

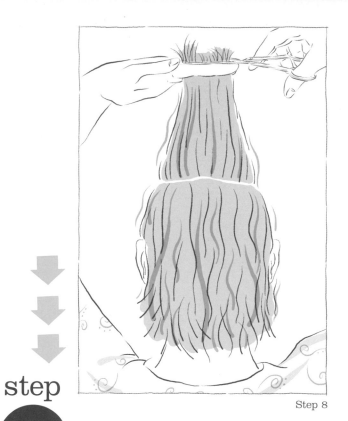

Step 8

step 8 CONTINUE CUTTING ONE-INCH SECTIONS USING THE PREVIOUS SECTION AS YOUR GUIDE. LOWER YOUR CHIN TO SEE THE BACK SECTIONS. IF YOU CANNOT SEE THE SECTIONS AT YOUR NECK, USE A HAND-HELD MIRROR TO LOOK AT THE SECTION, THEN GRASP IT IN A STRAIGHT LINE WITH TWO FINGERS. PUT THE MIRROR DOWN AND CUT JUST UNDER YOUR FINGERS. PUT THE SCISSORS DOWN AND USE THE HAND MIRROR TO CHECK THAT YOUR LINE IS STRAIGHT AND EVEN.

step 9 PART YOUR HAIR IN THE CENTER. ON ONE SIDE, MAKE A SLANTED VERTICAL PART IN FRONT OF YOUR EAR, CREATING A ONE-INCH SECTION.

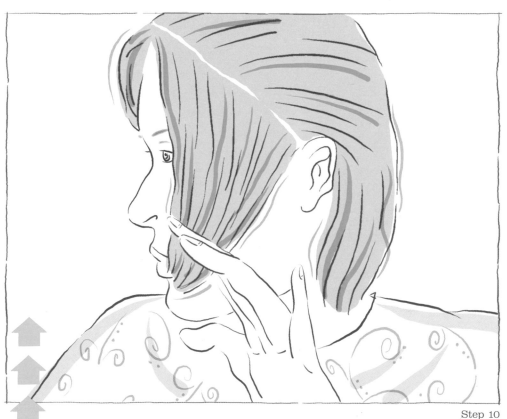

Step 10

step 10 COMB THIS SECTION FORWARD, AND GRASP IT BETWEEN TWO FINGERS WITH YOUR FINGERS PARALLEL TO THE PART.

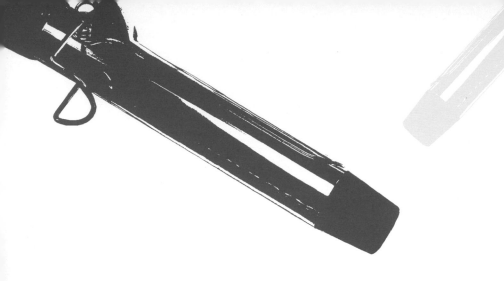

step
8

RELEASE THE SPOON, AND GENTLY PULL THE IRON OUT SIDEWAYS FROM THE ROLLED SECTION OF HAIR.

step
9

HOLD THE CURL WITH YOUR FINGERS 3–5 SECONDS THEN LET GO AND ROLL ADDITIONAL SECTIONS UNTIL ALL YOUR HAIR IS CURLED.

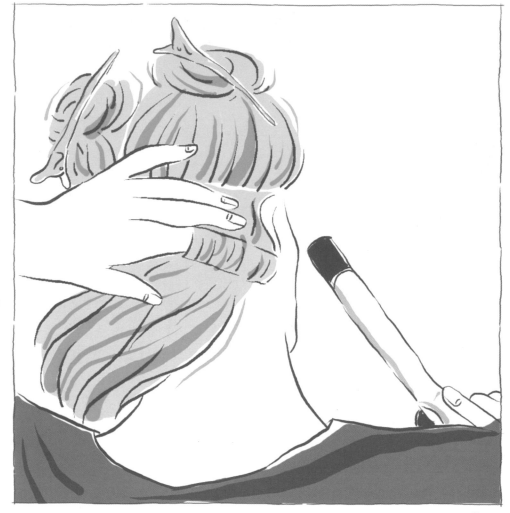

Step 9

step 11

CUT JUST UNDER YOUR FINGERS, USING THE FRONT SECTION YOU HAVE ALREADY CUT AS YOUR GUIDE.

step 12

CONTINUE MAKING ONE-INCH, SLANTED VERTICAL SECTIONS, COMBING THEM FORWARD BEFORE YOU CUT TO MATCH YOUR GUIDE. THE LAYERS WILL BE LONGER AS YOU MOVE TOWARD THE BACK OF YOUR HAIR.

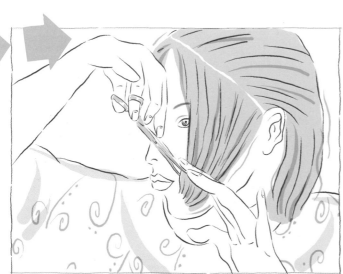

Step 11

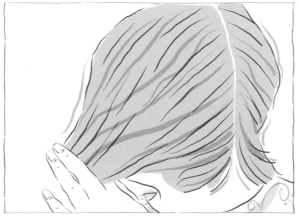

Step 12

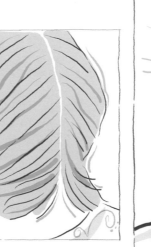

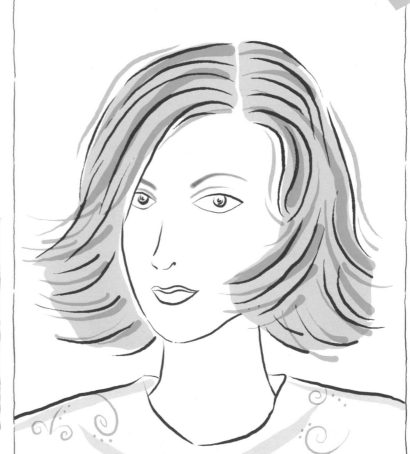

Final layered cut

step 13

REPEAT ON THE OPPOSITE SIDE TO FINISH.

step

7

HOLD THE IRON IN PLACE FOR THREE
TO FIVE SECONDS.

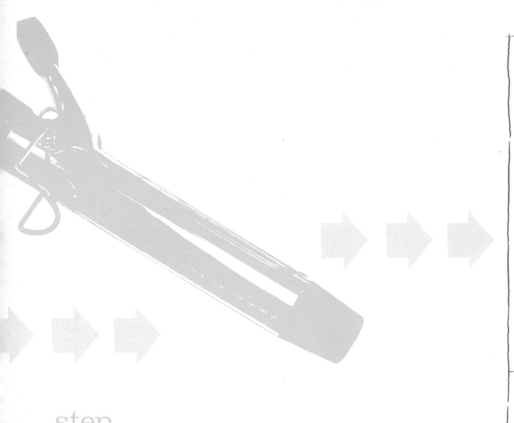

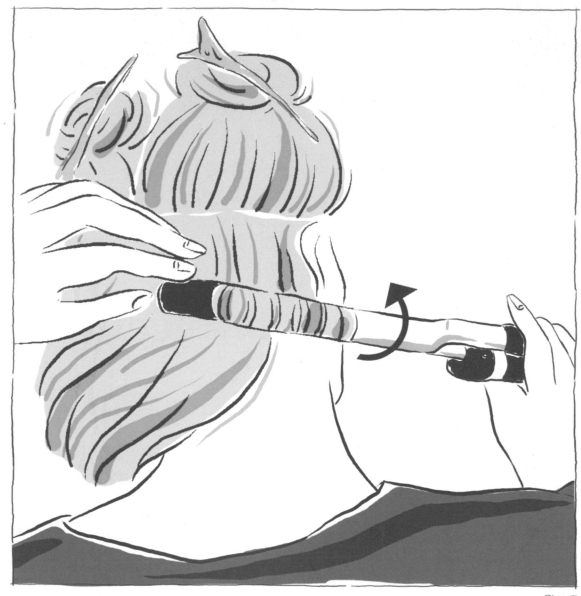

Step 7

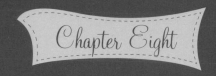

Chapter Eight

"ONCE YOU'VE HAD CHEMOTHERAPY, THERE IS NO SUCH THING AS A BAD HAIR DAY."

—Liz Tilberius

THE QUICK LAYERED CUT

Layering can make hair more versatile and give it more movement, and it works for both straight and curly hair. We have discovered a very easy way to layer your hair. Though it may seem like a bizarre way to cut hair, this method really does work!

One word of caution: be careful to center the rubber band exactly, or the sides will not be even. As for length, remember that the top will be as long as the distance from your hairline to the cut, and the same is true for the back.

step 1

DRY AND COMB THROUGH YOUR HAIR.

step 2

PICK UP A SECTION OF HAIR WITH ONE HAND.

step 3

COMB THE SECTION, AND PICK UP THE CURLING IRON.

step 4

CLAMP THE IRON WITH THE MOVABLE PART, CALLED THE SPOON, ABOUT AN INCH FROM THE END OF YOUR HAIR. TO CURL YOUR HAIR UP, CLAMP THE IRON WITH THE SPOON ON THE UNDERSIDE OF YOUR HAIR; TO CURL YOUR HAIR UNDER, CLAMP WITH THE SPOON ON TOP.

step 5

SLIDE THE CURLING IRON DOWN TO THE END OF THE SECTION, CATCHING ALL THE ENDS.

step 6

QUICKLY ROTATE THE CURLING IRON EITHER OVER OR UNDER YOUR HAIR, PICKING UP THE ENTIRE SECTION OF HAIR AS YOU ROLL. AVOID TOUCHING YOUR SCALP WITH THE IRON.

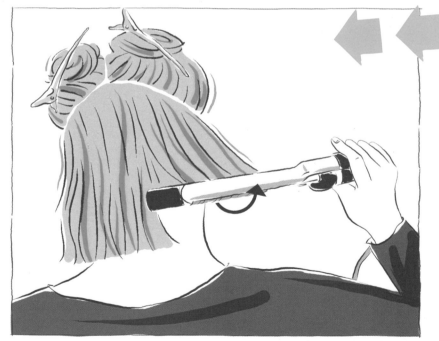

Step 6

step **1** WET YOUR HAIR, AND BEND OVER SO YOUR HEAD IS UPSIDE DOWN.

step **2** COMB YOUR HAIR INTO A PONYTAIL ON THE CROWN OF YOUR HEAD.

step **3** SECURE IT WITH A RUBBER BAND.

step **4** HOLD THE PONYTAIL STRAIGHT UP.

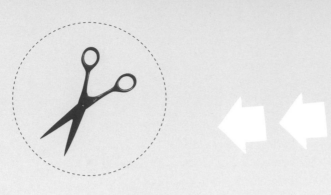

The Ironing Technique

In the past, the flat iron, curling iron and blow-dryer were available only to professionals because of the potential of these instruments to damage hair. Today there are a variety of curling irons and flat irons available in the consumer market, and they now have safety features. You can buy a flat iron or a curling iron in several price ranges, with particular features and materials determining price. Cheaper irons are made of metal, and higher-quality irons are ceramic and tourmaline, which conduct heat more evenly. Heating devices on better models give you more control and make it much less likely you'll burn your hair. As with any device, follow the manufacturer's instructions carefully so you don't burn your hair, scalp or skin.

CURLING IRON

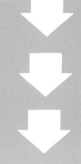

The curling iron goes back hundreds of years and used to be heated over a fire or on the stove. (Can you imagine how often ladies were scorched, or how many times whole chunks of their hair were burned off?) Results were often a dry and unruly frizz. Today curling irons are electric, and new ones are cordless. You can even buy a curling iron that folds up to be carried in your purse.

Use a curling iron instead of the old plastic or metal-and-mesh hair rollers. It is fast and gives you an instant set—without waiting, sleeping on rollers or sitting under a salon hair dryer.

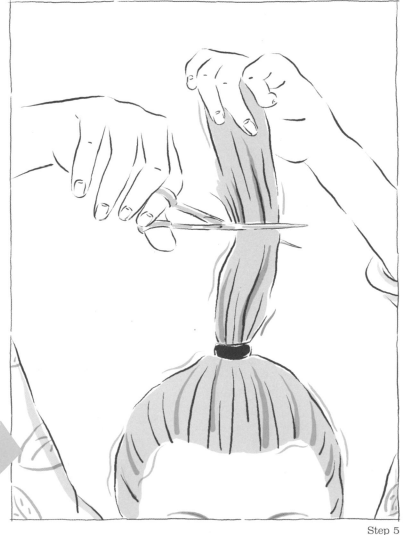

Step 5

5 CUT OFF THE END OF THE PONYTAIL. (THE LENGTH WILL BE DETERMINED BY HOW CLOSE YOUR CUT IS TO THE RUBBER BAND.)

step

6 REMOVE THE RUBBER BAND, SHAKE YOUR HEAD, AND YOU'VE GOT AN INSTANT LAYERED CUT!

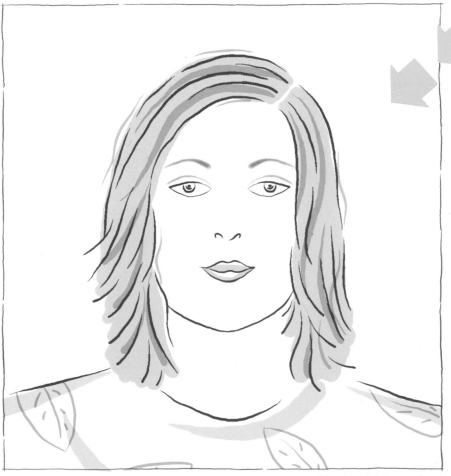

Final quick layered cut

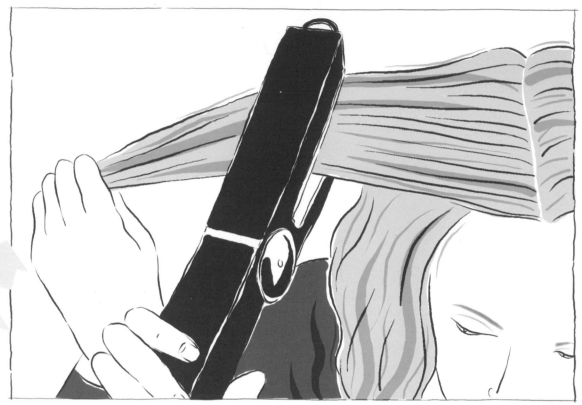

Step 5

step

5 CONTINUE WORKING ON EACH SECTION OF HAIR, FROM THE BOTTOM UP, UNTIL ALL YOUR HAIR IS IRONED.

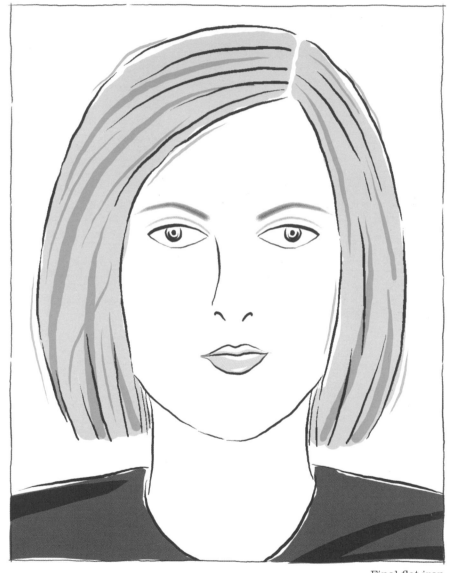

Final flat iron

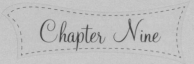

Chapter Nine

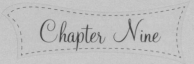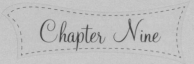

"MARGE SIMPSON'S BLUE BEEHIVE HAIRDO . . .
WAS INSPIRED BY A COMBINATION OF MY OWN
MOTHER'S HAIRSTYLE IN THE 1960S AND,
OF COURSE, **THE BRIDE OF FRANKENSTEIN.**"

—Matt Groening,

The New York Times Magazine, July 22, 2007

TIPS FOR DRYING AND STYLING

After washing and conditioning, towel dry your hair, removing as much water as possible. (Remember, blot your hair, don't rub.) This enables your styling products to be more effective, because they won't be diluted by water in your hair.

If you use gel or mousse, apply the recommended amount with your fingertips to your roots first, then work it into the rest of your hair. This gives you maximum control at the scalp, where you most want it.

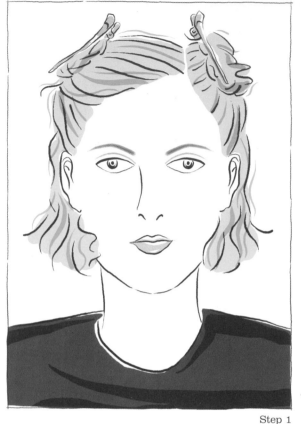

Step 1

step

1 SECTION THE TOP HALF OF YOUR HAIR AND CLIP IT ON TOP OF YOUR HEAD.

step

2 BEGIN AT THE BACK OF YOUR HEAD, AT THE NAPE OF YOUR NECK. COMB THIS SECTION TO REMOVE TANGLES AND MAKE IT SMOOTH. WORK WITH SMALL, MANAGEABLE SECTIONS, NO MATTER THE TEXTURE OF YOUR HAIR.

step

3 PLACE THE FLAT IRON ACROSS THE SECTION OF HAIR, WITH THE COMB EDGE NEXT TO YOUR SCALP, TEETH FACING AWAY.

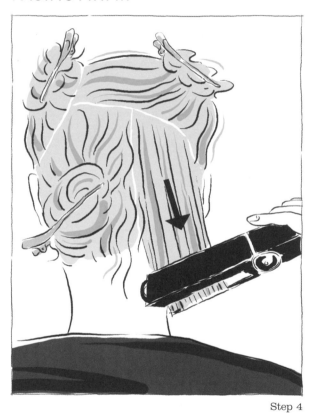

Step 4

step

4 GENTLY PULL THE IRON DOWN THE LENGTH OF YOUR HAIR, FROM YOUR SCALP THROUGH THE ENDS.

HOW TO
BLOW-DRY YOUR HAIR

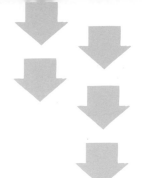

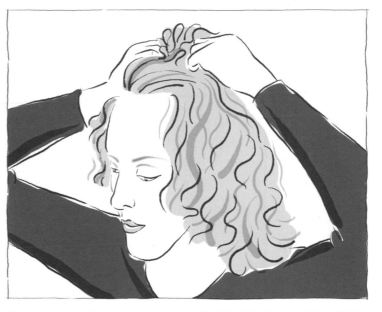

You can create a professional-looking hairstyle by using your blow-dryer properly. Using the right technique is important to styling your hair perfectly and avoiding damage to your hair from too much heat. The steps are not difficult and will give you great results.

It is essential to remove as much moisture from your hair as possible before blow-drying. Too much heat damages hair, but there are smoothing products on the market that coat the hair to help minimize damage. You can dry curly hair with a diffuser, which sometimes comes as an attachment with a blow dryer. Manipulate your hair with one hand while aiming the blow-dryer with the other.

Tips to Air-Dry Your Hair

* Overprocessed hair, damaged hair and curly hair should be air-dried. Blow-drying contributes to already damaged hair and makes it frizzy.

* After applying a styling product, comb your hair.

* Pinch, scrunch and push your hair, manipulating it into the shape or style you want.

* For a straight style, comb your hair and allow it to dry.

FLAT IRON

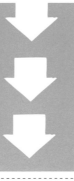

The flat iron does just what its name implies: it irons your hair flat and straight. The good thing about flat irons is they straighten without chemical treatments that can harm the structure of your hair and remove body and shine.

Flat irons are available wide and narrow. Use the narrow iron for short hair, and the wide one for medium and long hair. A good flat iron will have teeth on one side. This built-in comb frees up one hand. Inexpensive flat irons do not have a comb edge, making them less safe and more difficult to use. The curlier your hair, the more time it will take to iron it straight.

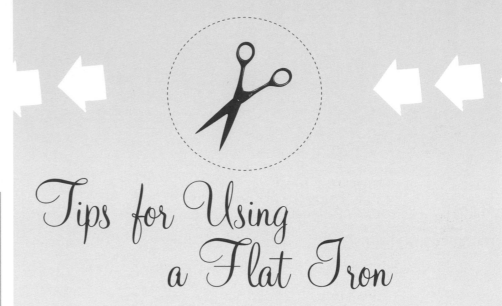

Tips for Using a Flat Iron

* Use a flat iron on dry hair only.

* It is important to place the comb edge of the flat iron toward your scalp, with the teeth facing away from your head, so you do not burn yourself. Use the flat iron by placing it across the section of hair at your scalp, and gently pull the iron from your scalp through the ends of your hair.

* Iron your hair in small, manageable sections, no matter the texture of your hair.

Tools for styling and drying

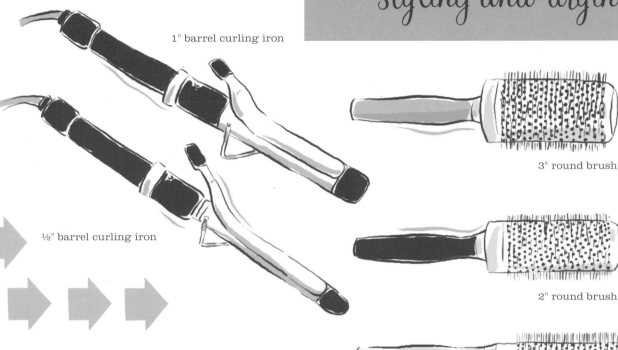

1" barrel curling iron

½" barrel curling iron

3" round brush

2" round brush

1" round brush

Vent brush

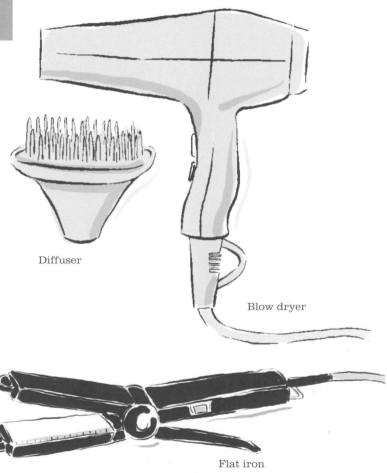

Diffuser

Blow dryer

Flat iron

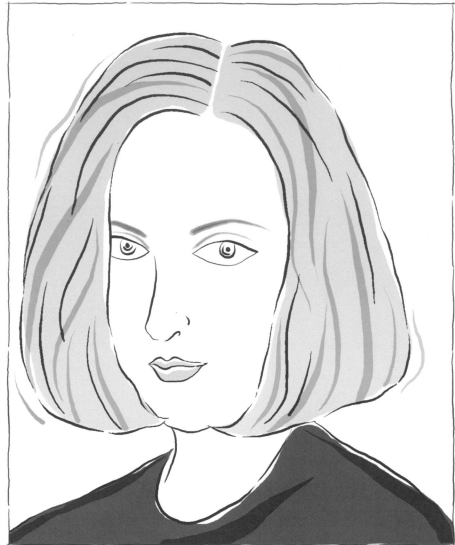

Final blow-dry

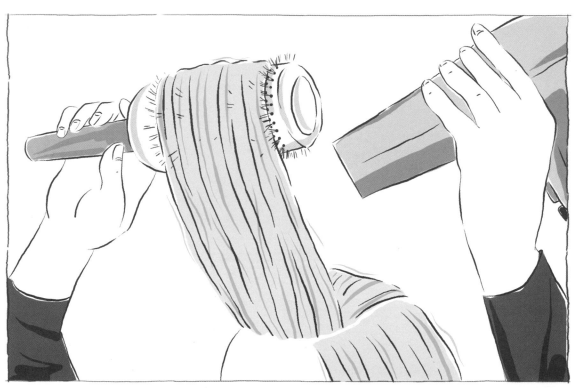

Step 6

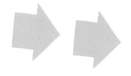

step

1 SECTION THE TOP FRONT OF YOUR HAIR AND CLIP IT OUT OF THE WAY.

step

2 BEGIN WITH THE BACK, BOTTOM SECTION. USE A VENT BRUSH FOR DRYING AND GETTING MORE AIR INTO YOUR HAIR, OR A ROUND BRUSH FOR SMOOTHING AND STYLING.

step

3 HOLD THE DRYER AT LEAST THREE INCHES ABOVE YOUR BRUSH TO AVOID BURNING YOUR HAIR OR SCALP, AND LAY THE BRUSH ON YOUR SCALP.

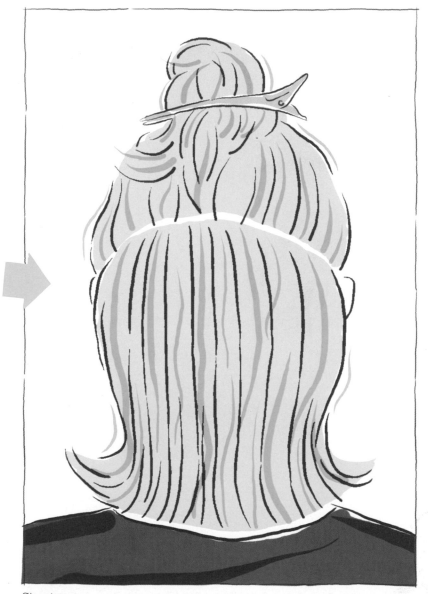

Step 1

step

4 ROLL THE BRUSH UNDER, GRABBING THE HAIR, AND GENTLY PULL THE BRUSH DOWN, FROM THE ROOTS TO THE ENDS.

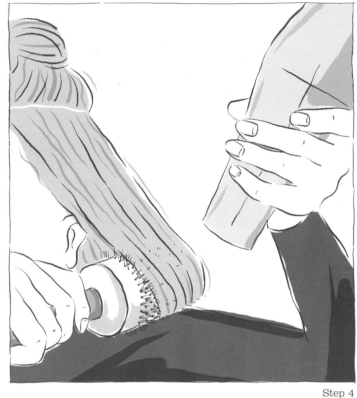

Step 4

 step

5 WHEN THE BOTTOM IS DRY, REPEAT THE PROCESS ON SIDE SECTIONS.

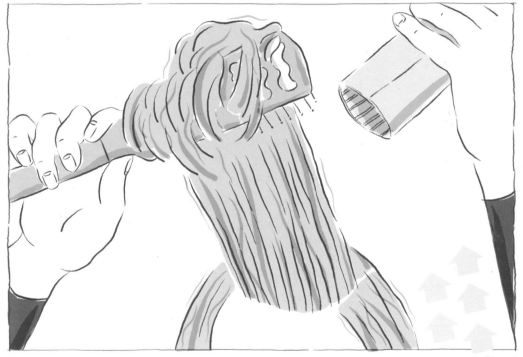

Step 6

 step

6 TO FINISH, PULL UP THE TOP SECTION A PIECE AT A TIME, AND BRUSH AND BLOW-DRY BY PULLING UP AND AWAY FROM YOUR SCALP, FROM YOUR ROOTS TO THE ENDS.